Cleanse
Your System

Find inner health through a unique
purification programme

Amanda Ursell

Thorsons
Directions for Life

For my parents and for Stuart

The author would like to thank Warner Wellcome for the use of data from their NOP survey on indigestion, in Chapter 9.

Thorsons
An Imprint of HarperCollins*Publishers*
77–85 Fulham Palace Road,
Hammersmith, London W6 8JB

Published by Thorsons 1999

1 3 5 7 9 10 8 6 4 2

© Amanda Ursell 1999

Amanda Ursell asserts the moral right to
be identified as the author of this work

Text illustrations by Peter Cox

A catalogue record for this book
is available from the British Library

Printed and bound in Great Britain by
Mackays of Chatham plc, Chatham, Kent

Contents

—— 1 ——
The Digestive System

Perhaps the best way to start this book is by telling you what it is *not* about. First, it is not about to start recommending you organize 10 colonic irrigation sessions to manually wash out your insides. Nor will it demand that you to start following some mad detoxification plan which leaves you starving in the mistaken belief that such emptiness must by implication be cleaning you out. Instead, *Cleanse Your System* is about understanding the reality of what goes on in your digestive system on a daily basis. By looking at what and when we eat, and how our emotional and psychological well-being play very direct roles in our digestive health, we learn to discover how to cleanse and calm our digestive systems – naturally.

The Sensitive Gut

Physically, your digestive tract is really just one long tube which is surrounded by muscles. This tube takes on different shapes and roles as it makes its way through the body from the mouth down into the throat, the stomach, on into the small and large intestine and finally to the rectum and anus.

This muscular tube cannot function on its own. To be able to break large pieces of food into smaller ones, mix them with various enzymes and acids, kill off the harmful bacteria and bugs we eat in our food, dispose of waste material and, finally, allow the absorption of useful nutrients into the bloodstream ... there needs to be a very efficient Commanding Officer.

The digestive system's CO comes in the form of its very own nervous system, known as the Enteric Nervous System or ENS. The

ENS communicates with the rest of the body and our brains via a huge and complex set of nerves (almost as many as in the brain itself). This means that what is going on in the gut affects our brain, and equally, what is going on in our brain affects our gut.

In practice this means the gut can tell the brain what to do and how to behave, and the brain can have direct effects on telling the gut what to do. Take the fact that simply looking at and smelling an appetizing meal can stimulate the flow of saliva. What has happened to elicit this response is that your senses of sight and smell have stimulated the brain. The brain has then sent a message to the ENS to tell it food is on its way and to start producing saliva in the mouth and acid in the stomach to get in preparation for the food which it believes is about to arrive.

Then there is the situation where the gut's nervous system tells the ENS something and the brain responds. For example, once some food such as meat enters the small intestine, the ENS sends a message to the brain telling it that some protein-breaking enzymes need to be released. The brain sends a message back to the gut which stimulates the release of some of the appropriate enzymes.

Digestion – What the Process Involves

Never before in history have we consumed such a huge array of different foods and drinks, and never before have we done so at such an extraordinary pace of life.

Each day we ask our digestive systems to deal with the processing of a huge variety of chemical substances, from the useful nutrients in foods and drinks to unfriendly bacteria and viruses and non-nutrient material which must be expelled from the system. Each section of the system has very distinct functions, and in turn suffers very distinct problems when things get out of kilter.

For much of the time we are blissfully unaware that our digestive systems are just getting on with the daily grind of transforming everything that enters our mouths into useful small-sized nutrients which can be absorbed, rendering harmful substances safe or separating out what is not needed and disposing of it as waste, either in our urine or stools.

These extraordinarily complex processes are, as already described, under the influence of the ENS and brain, along with quite a few chemical messengers known as hormones.

These processes are taking place all the time. We expect our digestive systems to keep on processing everything we throw at them without complaint.

That sometimes things go wrong – perhaps we suffer with a bout of heartburn, some trapped wind or something more problematic and long-term like Irritable Bowel Syndrome – is not surprising. There comes a point when the mix, quantities and pace at which we eat and drink can send our digestive systems into turmoil. At this point they start to rebel, letting us know in no uncertain terms that it is time for a break, time to think about restoring some balance and helping ourselves to a calmer, more peaceful internal existence.

— 2 —
The Mouth

Undoubtedly the most enjoyable part of eating and drinking occurs in the mouth, where food and drink first enter the body. It's here that we experience the textures and flavours that register as being pleasurable in the brain.

Just the sight and smell of food stimulate the brain to tell the nerves of the gut to begin producing saliva from the many salivary glands which line the inside of the mouth and cheeks. Once the flow has started and you actually get a delicious morsel into your mouth, the sheer mechanical action of physically chewing food stimulates further saliva production.

This is where the need for a good clean digestive system begins and where, if it is not achieved and maintained, poor digestion starts. A copious flow of saliva is crucial not only to the chewing and swallowing of food, but also to the cleanliness and condition of the teeth and gums. Tooth decay and gum disease are surprisingly common reasons for indigestion, and a lack of saliva increases the risk of both. Poor standards of oral cleanliness can also be responsible for bad breath, which immediately gives others the impression your digestive system could benefit from a quick spring-clean.

Saliva Production

In one day alone it is quite normal to produce over a litre (more than 1½ pints) of saliva. At rest we make about 0.5 ml (about ¼oz) per minute, which increases significantly on eating. Sucking a lemon (just the thought makes your mouth water), can cause a 100-fold rise in saliva flow.

A good flow of saliva physically helps clean the teeth and gums of chewed food by washing them away. The enzyme lysozyme, contained in saliva, helps to destroy potentially harmful bacteria, while the mucus coats chewed food so that when it moves on to be swallowed the oesophagus is protected from being scratched and damaged. Saliva also helps you to distinguish and enjoy flavours by dissolving components of foods which stimulate the taste buds.

A reduction in saliva production may be due to dehydration. Once you become thirsty it a sure sign that your body is already dehydrated and needs topping up with fluids as quickly as possible. This is a good survival mechanism because a dry mouth due to reduced saliva production brought on by dehydration is the strongest stimulus we have for searching out fluids to redress the imbalance.

Saliva flow is also severely restricted at times of severe mental effort and fear. Being uptight and worried when you eat can become a vicious circle, since a poor saliva flow makes eating less enjoyable, comfortable and tasty, which in turn can add to the stress of the experience.

That fear reduces salivary flow is well documented and has even been used as a crude test of a person's guilt or innocence in the 'Indian Rice Test'. A person unable to swallow dried rice was thought to be guilty on the grounds that fear prevents secretions. Goodness how many innocent people have been condemned on this basis. The fear of failing was probably enough to dry up any secretions they may have had.

Saliva and Tooth Decay

'Oh, I wish I'd looked after me teeth, and spotted the perils beneath,
all the toffees I'd chewed and the sweet sticky food, Oh, I wish I'd
looked after me teeth.'

So wrote Pam Ayres – a sentiment many of us echo as we endure the screeching of the dentist's drill. Keeping our teeth in good condition doesn't just save us from the horrors of the dental surgery, but aides digestion and promotes oral cleanliness.

Decay of the tooth occurs when remains of food eaten stick to the teeth and start forming plaque, a sticky substance which is an ideal breeding ground for the multiplication of bacteria which live in the mouth. The sugary substances in plaque are fermented by these bacteria, which produce acid – it is this acid which causes the enamel of the tooth to break down, causing decay right through into the softer dentine layers below. If the next layer of the tooth, the pulp, is also attacked, abscesses can form.

We have known for some time that the key to preventing tooth decay is avoiding sugary snacks between meals and brushing teeth regularly after eating to remove the vestiges of food which lead to plaque. Producing adequate saliva is also vital.

Saliva is naturally alkali and provides the safest environment in which the teeth can be bathed. Stimulating salivary flow after a meal helps to wash away bits of food and returns the mouth to its preferred alkali state. Chewing gum after a meal is a good way of increasing salivary flow, restoring a high pH and reducing the risk of decay.

The most effective chewing gums are those containing the natural sweetener xylitol. Made from the birch tree, xylitol has been shown in clinical research to reduce the risk of tooth decay through a variety of mechanisms.

First, the xylitol increases salivary flow above and beyond the capacity of normal gums, thus helping to raise pH and neutralize acids even more rapidly. Secondly, it inhibits the growth of the bacteria (*streptococcus mutans*) which grow on plaque. It is the only natural sweetener that has this property. Thirdly, it helps reduce decay by reducing the quantity of plaque produced in the mouth, making it less adhesive to teeth and thus easier to clean off. Finally, xylitol helps to remineralize areas of enamel which have already been attacked. Not only this, it keeps your breath fresh. Xylitol is added to Wrigley's Extra chewing gum, blue Smints and a variety of mouthwashes and toothpastes such as Boots Total Care toothpaste.

Other Roles of Saliva

In addition to the roles mentioned above, saliva also actually starts the breaking down of some nutrients. The enzyme amylase which is present in saliva begins the process of breaking down carbohydrates. Try chewing a piece of bread for a few minutes. As the salivary amylase enzymes start to work on the starch in the bread, they begin to turn into simple sugars which taste sweeter. The enzymes get to work on the surface of foods they come into contact with – so grinding food into very small particles in the mouth by chewing them thoroughly can promote this first stage of digestion. There is also a small amount of the enzyme which breaks down fat present in saliva.

Saliva is vital, too, for keeping the mouth moist to allow speech and oral comfort. A reduction in saliva production clearly has far-reaching consequences not just on the digestive processes and cleanliness of the mouth, but also on our ability to communicate easily and effectively.

Taking time to eat your food in peace and quiet, or at least giving yourself enough time to stop dashing and sit peacefully for a few minutes before you start, may help improve saliva flow if you are constantly on the go. Chewing slowly and thoroughly can help, as may mastering yoga breathing techniques. Trying to tempt people to eat who are down and have lost their appetite is not easy, but one way which may help is to stimulate saliva flow through good tastes and smells, hot, well-flavoured soups, an alcoholic apéritif or a mineral water with a splash of lime juice and a squeeze of lemon.

Halitosis

Typically caused by poor dental hygiene, and particularly by gingivitis, bad breath is a sure sign that your digestive system needs a spring clean. Try following the advice above. It is also worth making sure that your diet is rich in vitamin C – found in berries, citrus fruits, green peppers and dark green vegetables – plus beta carotene, found in carrots and dark red and green fruits and vegetables, to ensure any damaged and bleeding gums have the right nutrients to help rapid repair.

Also bear in mind that halitosis may also be due to disorders further down the digestive system, such as constipation and a change in gut bacterial flora. It is possible that the use of probiotics which restore good bacteria to the large intestine may help (see Chapter 6).

3
The Oesophagus

Once food has been chewed and mixed with saliva, it's time to swallow the masticated lumps into the first real 'tubular' part of the digestive tract, known as the oesophagus.

Swallowing is where the tongue springs into action. We swallow literally hundreds of times a day without giving a thought to just how complicated a process it is. In the way we learned during weaning, the tongue rises up and presses against the roof of the mouth. This forces the lump of food – or bolus as it's called in technical terms – into the back of the throat. This series of movements alone involves around 22 separate muscle groups. From here, rather like when you go to a fun fair and sit on the big dipper, once the starter switch has been pressed there's no going back.

The bolus is swept into the back of the throat (called the pharynx), an action that triggers nerves to tell the muscles surrounding the oesophagus to contract and relax in wavelike patterns. These pulsating movements carry the bolus like a raft on the rapids, downwards to the stomach.

The entire journey from mouth to stomach is remarkably quick, taking just four to eight seconds. Fluids travel even faster, whizzing through this part of the journey in one to two seconds.

To stop the bolus taking a wrong turning and shooting off into the windpipe instead of making its way on into the stomach, a small flap closes over the entrance to the windpipe to block it off. If you try to talk or inhale while swallowing, the protective mechanisms can be disrupted and short-circuited, with food getting into the breathing passageways. If this happens, frantic coughing is triggered, which is the body's way of trying to expel the food as quickly as possible and stop you choking.

Throughout its meandering course through the body, the digestive system is punctuated by valves and 'gateways'. The first of these is situated just above the entrance to the stomach. Known as the lower oesophageal valve, it too is closed off until it detects the approach of the bolus making its way down the oesophagus. As the bolus gets close to the top of the stomach, the muscular valve, acting as a gateway, opens, allowing the lump of food to continue on into the stomach, the bag-like storage tank of the digestive system.

The stomach environment is highly acidic and its lining is specially adapted to cope with the very corrosive nature of its contents. Other parts of the digestive tract lining the oesophagus are not acidic. It is quite normal for the valve which separates the oesophagus from the stomach to allow small amounts of the acidy contents to leak back up, they are then simply washed back into the stomach by regular swallowing of saliva. Some people suffer with severe reflux of their acidic stomach contents, which actually burns the oesophagus lining leading to the age-old cause of indigestion – heartburn. This is dealt with in more detail in Chapter 4.

Oesophageal Irritability

Another sensation which manifests itself as a pain in the chest, but is neither caused by heartburn nor serious heart problems, is oesophageal irritability, which may simply be caused by the muscular waves of the oesophagus getting out of kilter. Drinking very cold, very hot or carbonated drinks can all evoke odd and uncomfortable contractions. Even a loud noise like the sudden clapping of the hands can create this response in the oesophagus.

It has also been long suspected that an irritable oesophagus is related to emotional stress, anxiety or depression. Even setting someone tricky tasks in the school or work environment can be held responsible for sending the throat into uncomfortable spasm. Treating the root of the emotional stress may well help to relieve the physical indigestion it causes.

A Lump in the Throat

As well as an irritable oesophagus upsetting digestion, the feeling that you have a lump in your throat may have similar effects. It often comes between, rather that at, mealtimes, and tends to occur just below the Adam's apple level. It is noticeable during periods of strong emotions, often disappearing when you cry, but if left untreated can affect smooth swallowing and reduce the desire to eat.

It has been suggested that these lumps in the throat occur more often in tense people who swallow repeatedly, which creates a dry mouth and then the lump. Becoming 'choked up' with grief, disappointment or pride can also contract the throat muscles in an uncoordinated fashion, leading to further discomfort. Interestingly, a lump in the throat is often relieved by eating, drinking, having a good cry or seeking help to calm your underlying emotional tensions and worries.

Other Problems

A goitre occurs when the thyroid gland (situated in the throat) swells, leading to difficulties with swallowing as the goitre presses on the oesophagus, restricting its width. This is a problem that your doctor will need to treat.

The wide range of potential causes of digestive problems associated with the throat means that it is vital that any difficulties with swallowing be checked out by your doctor.

Action Plan

Dietary Advice

Once your doctor has identified the problem, advice on what to eat to keep nutrient intakes up is important. If swallowing needs to be relearned, then the help of both a speech therapist and a dietitian is invaluable.

Generally, the best foods to try if swallowing is a problem are those that are soft, need little chewing and will slip down easily. Chilled soft foods, like ice-cream, jellies, smooth yogurt, fromage frais, mousses and thick custards are good starting points. Slightly chilled foods are good, too, because they stimulate the swallowing reflex more easily than do warm ones. This is because there are more receptors that register cold temperatures at the back of the mouth than there are that register warm ones.

As swallowing improves, then you can move on to mixed-consistency foods.

Emotional Stress

Dealing with emotional stress is very important. See advice in Chapter 8.

Herbal Remedies

See Chapter 8.

4
The Stomach

The stomach is the point at which the digestive tract forms itself into a pouch and acts as a temporary reservoir. While it is possible to survive without a stomach, it does carry out some important digestive processes.

During the course of your life, your stomach learns to accept a bewildering array of lumps of food and a wide variety of drinks. A bolus (lump of food) may be hard, soft, acidic, alkaline, watery or solid. Whatever form each bolus takes when it enters the stomach, by the time it's ready to go on into the small intestine it needs to have been turned from a solid into a liquid, and that liquid needs to be of a consistent pH – in other words, not too acidic and not too alkaline. To ensure this, the stomach carries out several functions.

Like the rest of the digestive tract, the stomach is surrounded by lots of muscles. It can vary in shape a little from one person to another, but is generally a 'J'-shaped bag. In short, stout people it tends to run horizontally, whereas in tall, thin people the J is more vertical.

In either type of person, the stomach is surprisingly high up and not by the belly button, which is normally where we point toif complaining of stomach ache. When we are not eating (for example at night and for about four hours after the last meal), the stomach is relatively empty and looks like a deflated balloon, about 25 cm (10 in) long. In this state, it holds about 50 ml (2 fl oz), one third of a small yogurt pot. Once full, however, it can really expand, holding up to 4 litres (7 pints) of food and drink. This comes in handy for feast days, highdays and holidays when we usually overindulge. After a normal meal, it would contain more like 1.5 to 2 litres (2½ to 3½ pints).

One of the stomach's main roles is to put the muscles surrounding it into action. By contracting and relaxing, they set up a powerful churning motion, like a cement mixer, grinding and mixing its contents. Just as a builder would add water to thin a cement mix down, so the body secretes mucus and gastric juices, produced in copious quantities in the stomach wall. Nerves and hormones take the role of the builder controlling these additions, but these in turn are under the control of the foreman, the brain, which judges carefully how much of each needs to be added. The churning continues and the mucus and juices become thoroughly combined with the bolus.

The signal to start secreting, as we have seen, is given as soon as we see, smell or even think about food – a sort of advance party, letting the stomach know it's on standby. Once food and drink actually hit the stomach, more juices pour in from the walls of the stomach – partly in response to its physical presence, and partly due to the chemical make-up of the bolus it receives. The mucus that pours in is alkaline. It coats the stomach wall as well as mixing with the food and softening it up.

The juices contain three substances:

1. hydrochloric acid, which lowers the pH of the stomach environment and kills bugs
2. pepsin, which is an enzyme that helps digest protein
3. hormones, which control the contractions and movement of the muscular stomach.

The hydrochloric acid is extremely strong. When secreted, it immediately makes the stomach contents very acidic, with a pH of between 1.5 and 3.5 (neutral is pH 7). These acidic conditions are needed to help in the digestion of proteins and to kill off the many bacteria that enter the stomach in and with food and drink. Due to its low pH, hydrochloric acid is highly corrosive, apparently more so than the acid in a car battery, so that if the contents of the stomach were placed on a wooden table, they would bore their way through.

The acid clearly has a vital role, but the stomach wall has to be protected from it to avoid being damaged itself. Like most parts of the body when they are functioning properly, it has developed ways of getting round the potential problem. It does so in several ways. First, it has a thick coating of the alkaline mucus built up over it. Second, the cells of the stomach lining are very tightly cemented together, preventing gastric juices leaking into the tissues below. Third, if cells are damaged, they are quickly shed and replaced. The lining is completely shed and renewed every three to six days anyway to ensure that only fresh protective cells are in place.

The nerves and hormones that control the secretions and movements communicate directly with the brain. The brain controls the movements and secretions by detecting the physical presence and chemical compostion of food in the stomach via the nerves and hormones. The brain also affects the stomach's movements in response to external stimuli. Any form of anxiety, stress, emotional turmoil, fright or depression will be detected in the brain and exert their effect, through the nerves, on the stomach. In times of intense stress, for example, it's unlikely that you will feel the need to eat and so you can lose your appetite. The link between how we feel and the effect this has on all parts of the digestive tract should never be underestimated.

Certain components and nutrients in food and drink that enter the stomach can also directly affect the secretion of mucus and juice, and the valves at the top and bottom of the stomach.

Alcohol, aspirin and water are virtually the only substances that are absorbed directly from the stomach into the bloodstream – the rest must pass on into the small intestine.

Over a period of a few hours, the bolus will have gradually been broken down into a liquidy substance known as chyme. This has to pass out of the stomach and on into the first section of the small intestine, called the duodenum.

Problems with the Stomach

Heartburn

Heartburn is one of the commonest forms of indigestion, and the one people are usually describing when they complain of an 'acidy' taste in the throat and/or mouth. Heartburn occurs when the acid contents of the stomach spill back, past the sphincter into the gullet or oesophagus. On occasions, they may actually reflux right the way back and up into the mouth.

It's important to get the idea of reflux into perspective. Small amounts of reflux are actually perfectly normal and happen to most of us, most of the time. The muscular valve or gateway to the stomach allows some of the acidic mix of half-digested food to leak back out. It is in particularly susceptible people and those in whom large quantities seep out that the problem is both painful in the short term and a potential problem in the long term.

When you stop and think about it, it's hardly surprising that heartburn hurts. The stomach is equipped to deal with the acidic nature of its contents by having a thick, duvet-like coating of mucus to protect its surface. As we saw in Chapter 3, the oesophagus has no such protection. Swallowing saliva, which is alkaline, can help to neutralize the normal, small amounts of regurgitated acidic material, and the swallowing action itself helps to sweep these stomach contents back down to where they belong. If any is left, however, or reflux gets out of hand, the acid can literally start digesting the surface cells of the gullet and back of the throat. This is what causes the nerves to register pain.

Heartburn is most likely to occur when the valves at the top of the stomach and bottom of the gullet become weakened (see Figure 3). This is common in pregnancy when, it is believed, the extra levels of the hormone progesterone that are circulating have this weakening effect. Smoking is also thought to loosen the sphincter, as are certain drugs.

In other cases, the sphincter may be perfectly fit, but the pressure of, say, bending or lying down or lifting something heavy can overcome its ability to hold the stomach contents in and so leakage follows. Lying down soon after eating can lead to acid reflux, too. The stomach is physically tipped up and some of its contents forced past the valve and into the gullet.

Constipation, perhaps rather surprisingly, can cause reflux from the stomach into the gullet, too. When you strain to go to the toilet, the pressure builds up in the large intestine and has nowhere to go except back up the tract. The end result is that this pressure is relieved by the opening of the stomach valve, with reflux being the consequence. This is a good example of how something going wrong in one part of the gut can indirectly affect another part.

Extra pressure within the abdominal cavity has an adverse effect on sphincter strength as well. Pregnant women suffer not only from the effects of progesterone chemically weakening the sphincter, but from the foetus pushing the stomach and its contents up and, once again, forcing the stomach's contents up and out of the top of the intestinal sack. This is especially likely to occur during the last trimester and making changes to diet and lifestyle are the only steps that can be taken to help relieve this kind of heartburn (these are detailed below). The accumulation of fat in the abdominal cavity in both overweight and obese people has the same effect.

Certain foods can affect the strength of this gateway to the stomach. Fats, for example, seem to relax the muscle tone of the sphincter, as do coffee, alcohol, onions, garlic, peppermints and chocolates.

Very large meals – which not only fill the stomach to capacity, but also sit around for hours and take ages to digest – will often lead to reflux. This is usually an infrequent cause of problems, occurring at, say, Christmas, special parties and dinners and so on, and so shouldn't be unduly worried over. It is just nature's way of letting you know you've overdone it.

Heartburn is made worse in susceptible people by severe emotional upset. The brain-gut connection reacts, with fear, anxiety and anger stimulating reflux.

Above the stomach, there sits a big band of muscle separating the stomach from the lungs. Called the diaphragm, it is possible for the top part of the stomach to push up and through this muscular barrier, creating a hiatus hernia. Quite a few sufferers experience reflux and heartburn as a result of having a hernia.

In a few people, the refluxing of the stomach's contents into the gullet can lead to inflammation. Severe cases may result in bleeding, which, if it carries on over a period of time, can lead to anaemia. The inflammation, or oesophagitis as it's known, may eventually cause scarring and a narrowing of the gullet. This is obviously uncomfortable and may ultimately lead to cancer.

As you can see, it is vital that any serious refluxing is reported to your doctor, who may decide to investigate and look into things further. An investigation with an endoscope might be recommended, which involves swallowing a narrow tube – the endoscope – which has a camera and light in the end to enable the doctor to have a good look around and also take little tissue samples from the gullet to study under a microscope later.

There is a plethora of drugs and remedies available on prescription from the doctor or over the counter at the chemist's for heartburn. Equally, there are many positive dietary and lifestyle improvements you can make that can help to reduce the number and severity of attacks.

Dietary Advice

How and when you eat cannot be separated from the chemical composition of the food and drink itself in terms of the effects on your digestive system.

First of all, always try to make time to eat and drink and avoid, whenever possible, doing either when on the go. Sit down and leave yourself time, however short of it you are.

Chewing thoroughly is also important. It not only gets the digestive process off to a good start by thoroughly mixing in enzymes and turning food into small and easy-to-swallow pieces, it helps avoid the 'bolting' down of a meal or snack.

If you make yourself calm prior to eating and take the whole process at a more leisurely pace, your nervous system will calm down and produce less acid in the stomach.

Timings and Quantities

It's best to avoid huge influxes of food and drink at any one time to reduce the risk of overfilling the stomach. The stomach holds 1.5 litres (2½ pints) comfortably without becoming badly overextended. If too much is eaten at one go, the stomach becomes overfull, it cannot empty itself fast enough to clear it and reflux is likely.

This means it's important not to skip meals, only to overindulge several hours later. Small, regular intakes – such as a light breakfast, mid morning snack, lunch, mid-afternoon snack and finally a light evening meal – is the best pattern to adopt to avoid reflux and heartburn. It is vital that you leave time after your last meal of the day for the food to start moving from the stomach into the intestine – in other words, a good few hours before going to bed. The risk of *not* following such a rule is that, as soon as you lie down, the contents of the stomach move into the oesophagus by sheer virtue of gravity. So, why deliberately make things worse for yourself?

The Chemical Composition of Foods

Certain components of foods and drinks can actually weaken the sphincter at the top of the stomach.

Protein-rich meals seem to enhance the tone of the valve, making it tighter and, therefore, a better blocker. Good sources of protein include lean meat, poultry without the skin, fish (white and oily), eggs and reduced-fat dairy products, such as milk and cheese.

Fatty foods have quite the opposite effect. Meals and snacks rich in fat *relax* the sphincter, making reflux and therefore heartburn in susceptible people more likely. Most people in the West consume more calories than necessary from fats and would be well advised to reduce their totals for other health reasons. Diets rich in fat are more likely to lead to putting on weight. If high in saturated fatty acids, they can increase cholesterol levels in the blood and thus the risk of heart disease.

Fats have another action on the stomach that can make heartburn more likely. When a fat-rich bolus reaches the stomach, small bits of it are passed on into the top part of the small intestine. In this section, the duodenum, it is recognized that the fat content is high, which stimulates the release of a hormone called enterogastrin. This hormone acts as a messenger and tells the muscles of the stomach to slow down its contractions. With the movements of the muscles reduced, the mixing and grinding takes longer and food stays in the stomach for greater periods of time. In those who suffer refluxes, the time period over which it could occur is therefore increased as a fatty meal can remain in the stomach for up to four or five hours.

Cutting back on fat is important from a weight point of view, too. As mentioned, fatty diets tend to lead to weight gain. Gram for gram, fats contain twice the calories of carbohydrates and protein, so a teaspoon of fat such as butter, margarine or oil will provide 37 calories while a teaspoon of a protein food like lean beef will provide around 10. A fatty diet is therefore far more energy dense than one rich in carbohydrates and proteins. That is, many more calories are packed into a small quantity of fatty foods than are contained in carbohydrates and proteins.

It's easy to monitor the amount of fats we take in when we can actually *see* them. These so-called 'visible fats' are things like butter, margarines and oils. They are all virtually 100 per cent pure fat and are very high in calories. Much more of a problem are the fats lurking in foods, and in some cases drinks, that are well disguised. Looking on the packets of foods often gives the game away. If fats, oils, margarine or butter appear high up on the list of ingredients, then it is sure to contain a fair amount of them as ingredients are listed in order of the quantity used, with whatever there ismost of appearing first and whatever there is least of appearing last. There are many foods containing such hidden fats that, in theory, aren't a surprise. Biscuits and cakes, creamy foods and things that are fried are bound to be rich in fats. Sometimes the actual quantities they contain can be quite staggering though.

Hidden Fats in Foods

2 shortbread fingers	9 g (⅓ oz)
2 coconut cookies	5 g (⅙ oz)
2 lemon puffs	10 g (⅓ oz)
Original crunchy bar	7 g (¼ oz)

Cherry bakewell	7 g (¼ oz)
Apple pie	8 g (¼ oz)
Puff slice	12 g (½ oz)
Flapjack slice	6 g (⅕ oz)
Viennese whirl	13 g (½ oz)
Cheese and tomato pizza (200g)	20 g (¾ oz)
Pork pie	37 g (1⅓ oz)
Steak and kidney pie	22 g (¾ oz)
2 pork sausages	30 g (1 oz)
Cornish pasty	29 g (1 oz)
Sausage roll	16 g (½ oz)
Fish and chips	38 g (1⅓ oz)
Coleslaw (per 50 g/2 oz)	8 g (¼ oz)

Savoury snacks are an area to really watch. Most are based on potatoes or corn and are then fried. Both potato and corn are able to absorb large amounts of fats during frying, so will be literally dripping in calories.

Snack	Packet Size	Calories	Fat
Bombay mix	100 g (4 oz)	494	32 g (1 oz)
Potato crisps	30 g (1 oz)	160	11 g (⅓ oz)
Peanuts	25 g (1 oz)	143	12 g (½ oz)
Trail mix	100 g (4 oz)	495	31 g (1 oz)
Les mignons	100 g (4 oz)	515	35 g (1¼ oz)
Tortilla chips	100 g (4 oz)	490	25 g (1 oz)

Other foods to be aware of are those with added cheese. Cheese is an excellent source of protein and calcium. However, it is also high in fats, the amount varying depending on the type, so if cheese is sprinkled over something such as a pizza or jacket potato, the totals of fat and calories will shoot up.

Returning to the valve. This little muscular ring at the entrance to the stomach is susceptible to chemicals in food over and above just proteins and fats. Perhaps one of the most surprising of these is peppermint. It is fairly traditional to serve mints after a meal as they do aid digestion further down the tract. In those who are prone to gastric reflux, the best advice is to pass on them. The peppermint acts as a smooth muscle relaxant. When it comes into contact with the sphincter, therefore, it will cause it to relax and lose tone, making it easier for the stomach contents to leak back into the oesophagus.

Caffeine, found in coffee, tea and cola, has a similar effect, making the ritual of coffee and mints after a meal a complete nightmare for the refluxer. The amount of caffeine commonly found in just one or two cups of coffee has been shown to slightly relax the valve just 30 to 45 minutes after drinking it.

If the mints are coated in chocolate, this will truly seal your fate as chocolate is yet another substance that will relax the valve acting as the stomach's gatekeeper. The effect of chocolate on the valve may be due to its methylxanthine content. Methylxanthines are related to the caffeine family of substances. Drinking hot chocolate, even the reduced fat versions, before going to bed is also a habit best discouraged if heartburn is a problem.

Alcohol weakens the muscular valve, too, so, again, go easy, and a liqueur is the last the thing you need after a big meal.

Some evidence suggests that onions and garlic have adverse effects on valve tone, too, so it is worth testing the theory out and seeing if reducing them in the diet works for you.

Concentrated solutions of sugar or salt may directly irritate the oesophageal membranes that have already been damaged by reflux. This may explain why some fruit juices and tomato juice are poorly tolerated. The high sugar concentration may be more irritating than the acid content. Spicy foods can also have a direct, negative effect on the already damaged areas.

Action Plan

Heartburn due to reflux is painful and distressing and eventually will take the enjoyment out of eating and drinking. Reduce the risks of reflux by following the simple rules below.

Plan Your Meals

Make time for your meals, however little spare you have, by setting aside a calm 20 minutes to eat and drink. Eating on the hoof can be a false economy where time is concerned if following the meal you are then debilitated by uncomfortable refluxing.

One way of slowing down is to use a different method of eating to the one you normally use. Try chopsticks, for example. If you are not practised in using them, they will definitely slow you down, although, of course, this isn't very practical when you are out in restaurants or with friends.

Chew slowly. Start by training yourself to chew everything 40 times before swallowing. It has a remarkably calming effect and presents food to your stomach in a more digestible form.

Eat little and often. Plan your day so that you don't have any heavy meals at night time. If you get peckish in the evenings, then stick to light fruits or yogurts.

Avoid cigarette smoking, especially in the evening before going to bed, as this weakens the valve to the stomach.

Get the overall balance of your diet right by including the correct amounts of starchy carbohydrates, proteins, fats and sugars.

Drinks

As a rule, try to avoid coffee and strong tea, as well as hot chocolate and cola drinks. Decaffeinated versions of tea, coffee and cola can be found, but, still, go easy as they do contain some caffeine.

Alternatives include drinks such as Barley Cup and Caro, herb teas and herb-based soft drinks, such as Purdys and Aqua Libra, and you can't go wrong with straightforward still water.

Intakes of alcohol do need to be controlled and kept to a minimum because, as we have seen, it is able to loosen the stomach valve.

Gastritis

Spices contain volatile oils, which are also capable of physically irritating the stomach lining. This is a purely direct physical reaction, unlike the chain of events set in motion by caffeine production. Hot curries, chillies and chilli sauces used in Mexican and other foods and some drinks, like spicy tomato juices, Virgin and Bloody Marys are best avoided. A very hot chilli or curry dish that contains a blend of pungent spices can literally bore a hole in the stomach lining.

Foods to Eat

- dairy products, such as milk, milky drinks, yogurts, fromage frais, cottage cheese, custards and rice puddings
- foods rich in soluble fibre, which includes porridge oats and stewed apples and pears
- soft, non-acidic fruits, including melons, guavas, papayas and apricots – both dried and rehydrated
- Root vegetables, including potatoes, turnips and parsnips

Foods to Avoid

- spicy dishes, such as curries, if you are not used to them
- chillies in dishes and drinks

Drinks to Take

- skimmed milk-based drinks, using coffee and tea substitutes
- vegetable juices not based on tomato, such as carrot
- water

Drinks to Avoid

- fruit juices
- tomato juice
- coffee
- tea
- cola drinks

Burping and Belching

Burping and belching, like clothes and food, are subject to fashions and trends. Considered a sign of appreciation after a good meal back in Tudor times, burping after a dinner party nowadays would offend and embarrass the other people there. So, burping and belching are now largely consigned unceremoniously to the indigestion category as something we want to avoid.

Both long, hearty belches and short, sharp burps are, whatever your attitude towards them, a perfectly normal part of the digestive process, as they help to expel air that has collected in the stomach. While a baby is growing in the womb, the digestive tract is free from air. Once born, from the first inhalation of breath, the system gradually takes in air, especially when feeding, making it inevitable that the baby will need to burp.

When we need to burp, this indicates that quite a bit of air has accumulated in the stomach. This can produce symptoms varying from mild discomfort to quite unbearable cramping pain. Releasing the air from the stomach, up into the oesophagus and out of the mouth gives almost immediate relief.

Once again, eating habits, smoking and lifestyle all affect the quantity of air swallowed and produced. If air were water, straightforward swallowing involves taking down about a teaspoonful. Eating quickly, chatting, laughing, smoking and consuming carbonated drinks all increase the quantity of air swallowed and the necessity to bring it back up as burps or belches.

Dietary Advice

The advice for belching is very similar to that for bloating. It is especially important in this case to eat slowly and not to eat and talk at the same time as this encourages large amounts of air to be swallowed along with the food.

Chewing gum is also not recommended, and avoid carbonated drinks.

Eat and drink slowly, making time for both. Doing either quickly will lead to swallowing large amounts of air and so aggravate belching problems.

An infusion of ginger can help relieve the need to belch. Try pouring boiling water into a cup containing a teaspoon of freshly grated ginger root and leave the mixture to stand for five minutes before straining off the liquid and drinking it. Alternatively, you could try chewing a ginger biscuit.

If you don't suffer from reflux, sucking a strong peppermint may also help relieve the problem.

Gently rubbing the stomach can help dislodge any trapped wind in the stomach, as can bending down from the waist or taking gentle exercise.

Food Diaries

If you suffer regularly from belching, and, indeed, flatulence, dietary culprits can often be identified by keeping a food diary. This involves writing down everything you eat and drink over a five or seven-day period. It is necessary to record the times the food and drink were consumed and how you felt at the meal – whether it was rushed, whether you sat and had it quietly and so on. You also then need to record the time and severity of any symptoms that follow.

Over the course of a week, it should be possible to identify whether certain foods, drinks or situations are regularly precipitating the problem. It may seem like a chore, but this is a proven method of identifying causes of problems. For instance, a lot of people who suffer migraines complete such diaries to help identify trigger factors for their severe and debilitating headaches.

Gastric Ulcers

Ulcers can occur in the stomach, which account for about 20 per cent of all ulcers, or, much more commonly, in the duodenum, which make up the remaining 80 per cent.

Stomach, or gastric, ulcers must be taken seriously. They can be the next step on from gastritis, which is when local areas of the lining of the wall of the stomach are eroded. Unlike gastritis, ulcers don't just occur due to an overproduction of, or imbalances in, acid production. Gastric ulcers can be single or multiple, acute or chronic, large or small. They can appear, heal and leave you in peace then re-emerge again suddenly. The acid production is often normal or even reduced in people who suffer stomach ulcers, so the problem seems more likely to stem from the mucus not being able to withstand the normal acidic conditions in the stomach. This might be because it has been under constant attack from irritants, such as aspirin and alcohol.

Gastric ulcers can cause discomfort once in a while or can, at the other end of the spectrum, lead to excruciating pain if the ulcer perforates and penetrates into surrounding tissues or organs. Pain associated with stomach ulcers usually sets in around one to one and a half hours after eating.

There is no strong consensus on 'natural' causes of ulcers. They do seem, however, to run in families, occur in people with type O blood and in those who push themselves hard at work and often at play as well.

There is a growing consensus in the medical world that a large number of ulcers are caused by an infective agent, a bacteria called *Helicobacter pylori*. Work carried out in Australia by Dr Barry Marshall and his team of researchers revealed that, on average, *H. pylori* is present in 65 per cent of patients with stomach ulcers and 85 per cent with duodenal ulcers. However, *H. pylori* is present in the stomachs of many people who don't have ulcers, so the link between this bacteria and ulcers is not quite clear. It could be that people carrying *H. pylori* get ulcers by an unfortunate quirk of their biochemical make-up. If this is so, it would fit in with the observation that ulcers tend to affect members of the same family.

It is known that certain drugs used for arthritis – non-steroidal anti-inflammatory drugs (NSAIDs) – can, unfortunately, lead to perforation of the stomach wall, as can large, continued doses of aspirin.

Ultimately, drugs will probably be needed to heal the ulcer. However, diet and lifestyle can contribute to the relief of symptoms and help in the healing process.

Dietary Advice

The good news is that the old-fashioned diets of bland foods based on milk and milk puddings and strict dietary programmes have not been proven to be effective in the treatment and management of gastric ulcers, so there is no need to restrict yourself to these kinds of uninspiring choices.

For years, it was believed that milk somehow neutralized an 'acid stomach'. Tests have shown that milk has only a passing neutralizing effect on gastric acids and is actually rapidly followed by a rise in acidity. So, it seems that those who spent long periods on a bland diet of white fish, mashed potato and milky drinks did so in vain. Such a regimen *doesn't* help to heal ulcers.

There are some general guidelines which can be followed as part of a modern gastric diet:

- meals should be small, frequent and regular
- very hot or very cold foods should be avoided as they encourage air to be swallowed, which aggravates the problems
- fried foods should be avoided
- leave out any pickles, black pepper, vinegar, spices and mustard
- avoid tea, coffee, colas, cold remedies with caffeine and alcohol, which all stimulate acid production
- according to herbalists, liquorice has a soothing action on mucous membranes and is often given to help treat ulcers (it can be taken as a drink by pouring hot water over a liquorice root and allowing to simmer for 15 minutes).

While consumption of alcohol can rarely be identified as the cause of an ulcer, wine and drinks with 5 per cent or more alcohol are potent stimulants of gastric acid secretion and should therefore be avoided by those with ulcers.

Caffeine again rears its head. Like alcohol, most studies have revealed that while it doesn't *cause* ulcers, it can exacerbate pre-existing conditions. Tea has been shown to have a similar effect after just 200 ml has been consumed, which is just a couple of mugs.

B_6 is a vitamin found in meat, milk, potatoes and other vegetables. Some ulcer sufferers have been found to have low levels of this vitamin circulating in the blood. It has been suggested that supplementing with B_6 vitamin could help in the healing of ulcers. The same is true of observational studies on gastric ulcer patients who have taken vitamin C supplements.

Foods rich in vitamin C include all citrus fruits, such as oranges and grapefruits and their respective juices, berries, like strawberries, raspberries and blackberries, kiwi fruit, peppers including red, yellow and green, green leafy vegetables, sweet potatoes, parsley and, in smaller amounts, parsley and ordinary potatoes.

Modest supplements of both vitamins B_6 and C could be considered, but check with your doctor before taking them.

Some research has shown that when laser therapy was given to a group of people with gastric ulcers, it was more effective when given together with vitamin E supplements.

Vitamin E is found in good amounts in wheatgerm oil, and other vegetable oils, wholegrain cereals, eggs, dark green leafy vegetables, such as spinach and dark green cabbage, and sprouts. Avocados are also a good source, as are blackberries.

Taking zinc sulphate supplements has also been looked into and seems to have a degree of success in some people with gastric ulcers. Note, though, that it is easy to take too much zinc, so don't take this supplement without checking amounts with your doctor.

Oysters are the best, and unfortunately the most expensive, source of zinc. Red meat is the next best, however, with lean beef and lean pork boasting the highest amounts. Cheddar cheese is also rich in zinc, as are the dark meat from chicken, lentils, wholegrain cereals, rice and maize.

Work has also been carried out on the effect of essential fatty acids (EFAs) on gastric ulcers. Both those found in vegetable oils, such as sunflower, safflower and evening primrose, as well as those from oily fish, like salmon, tuna, mackerel, sardines, kippers and pilchards, have been indicated to have a positive effect.

It seems that the EFAs in the vegetable oils may enhance ulcer healing. The theory behind their role lies in the fact that EFAs are converted in the body into hormone-like substances known as prostaglandins. Various pieces of evidence indicate these prostaglandins may play a physiological role in protecting the gastric mucous membranes. Supplementing with EFAs in the form of evening primrose oil (Efamol) and fish oils may help protect against and treat ulcers.

There is some evidence that high-fibre diets may be of benefit – not in the healing process, but in delaying the time of another ulcer occurring. This is an area in which further study is needed, but, as a high-fibre diet is essentially a healthy way of eating and will help to provide the nutrients mentioned above, for example B_6, zinc and vitamins C and E, it is certainly worth following such a diet.

Foods rich in fibre include wholegrain breads, wholegrain cereals, like brown rice and pasta, and breakfast cereals such as bran flakes, All Bran, Weetabix, Shredded Wheat, porridge and muesli and granola. Pulses, vegetables and fruit are also good sources.

There is not enough proof from these research findings for dietitians to recommend particular strategies based on them to patients, but they are continuing areas of interest and more remains to be found out and confirmed.

5

The Small Intestine

After the stomach, the gut reverts to a tube shape, and this part of the digestive system is the small intestine. Only about 2.5 cm (1 in) wide, it's a staggering 2 m (6½ feet) long. This great length of tubing is carefully arranged in the region we usually refer to as our stomach – the space below the ribcage. If the intestines were stretched out rather than being neatly folded as they are, we would be a very tall race.

The small intestine is where the bulk of the digestive process takes place. The stomach has mechanically turned the food and drink into the liquidy chyme described earlier, and between it and the mouth has already started chemically breaking down proteins, carbohydrates and fats. The small intestine, though, is sitting in wait with a complete army of enzymes to continue the job. It is here where proteins are broken down into their smallest form, amino acids, carbohydrates to simple sugars and fats to fatty acids and glycerol. It is here also where essential vitamins and minerals in foods are absorbed into the blood to be carried off to perform various functions around the body.

Under the microscope, the wall of the small intestine looks like grass blowing in the wind. This is because the wall is formed into very fine finger-like projections known as villi. They are about a millimetre (less than ⅛ in) tall and feel velvety. Digested nutrients are absorbed through the wall of villi into little blood vessels which run inside them.

The villi increase the absorbtive surface of the small intestine enormously – yet another space-saving device. It has been estimated that the entire absorptive surface these villi provide is equivalent to 200 sq. m (239 sq. yards). That is, the floor space of an average two-storey house. If there were no villi, the small intestine would have to be even longer than it already is.

Intestinal juices, which contain some of the necessary breakdown enzymes, are secreted from the walls of the intestine in quantities of 1 to 2 litres a day. They pour into the intestine when the chyme leaves the stomach and enters the duodenum.

Enzymes are also secreted directly from the intestinal walls and from the pancreas – an organ that sits alongside the intestine and also secretes some enzymes. The pancreas is vital for another reason. The chyme from the stomach is still acidic at this point and must be made neutral so that it doesn't damage the intestine wall. The pancreas pumps alkaline juices into the intestine to effect this neutralization.

In addition to enzymes, the intestine receives a secretion from the gallbladder – another small organ situated close by. The gallbladder squirts in bile, which is a rather unpleasant-looking yellowy green liquid. This happens when the intestine registers that the chyme from the stomach is particularly fatty after a fat-rich meal has been eaten. The hormone cholecystokinin (CCK) acts as the messenger, racing from the intestine to tell the gallbladder to start firing. Bile is able to emulsify or homogenize fats. A good example of homogenization is homogenized milk, which has the fat evenly distributed throughout so that no cream line forms. This, essentially, is what bile does to fats in the intestine. It distributes them evenly, thus giving the fat-breaking enzymes a chance to get to work on them.

Food is moved down the tube by the muscles that surround it. They contract and relax rhythmically in a motion known as peristalsis. These little waves of movement gradually push the contents forwards and backwards, offering them up to the villi to be absorbed.

The end of the small intestine is blocked off from the start of the final section of the system – the large intestine – by another valve. Nerves and hormones tell the valve to open to allow undigested material from the meal and bacteria to move on into the large intestine. The valve is important not so much for letting the material through, but for stopping contents of the large intestine creeping back into the small intestine.

The small intestine, like the stomach, is wired up to the brain via a huge number of nerves. Thus, any stress, anxiety or worries can again be transmitted to the system and affect its functioning in very significant ways.

Duodenal Ulcers

These are ulcers that develop in the very first part of the small intestine and seem, unlike stomach, or gastric ulcers, to be aresult of overproduction of acid in the stomach. They canalso develop as a result of the stomach emptying too much ofits acidic contents into the duodenum in one go, and the duodenum having insufficient alkaline secretions present to neutralize them. The bacteria *H. pylori,* mentioned above, may play an important role in the development of duodenal as well as stomach ulcers.

Like gastric ulcers, duodenal ulcers occur when there has been erosion of the mucous membranes. They may be single or multiple, superficial or deep.

Duodenal ulcers seem to be strongly hereditary – probably because the overproduction of acid runs in families. They are far more common than stomach ulcers. The finger of blame can, once again, in part, be pointed at stress. This was seen clearly to be the case in London during the Second World War where the number of people with ulcers increased dramatically during the air raids. The theory goes that excessive nerve stimulation increased acid production, which led to duodenal ulcers developing. While air raids are a thing of the past, it's easy to see how the pressures of modern life could easily lead to a similar end result. Tight deadlines, frantic schedules, combining family responsibilities with work, bringing up children, financial and emotional worries, combined with other day-to-day problems can create untold stress.

Dietary Advice

Similar dietary guidelines apply for duodenal ulcers as stomach ulcers.

Researchers have tried treating duodenal ulcers with apple pectin (the substance in fruit that makes jam set). When patients were given around 12 mg a day, the pectin seemed to help prevent relapses. The researchers suggest that apple pectin could therefore be used as a form of treatment to help reduce the risk of recurring duodenal ulcers. This treatment is not widely used, however, and so should be talked through with your doctor.

A generally high-fibre diet may, as with stomach ulcers, help reduce the risk of further duodenal ulcers occurring. Research with patients who have duodenal ulcers has shown a dramatically lowered incidence of recurrence in those who follow such a diet, which, some researchers believe, could be because of the increased amount of chewing high-fibre diets require. The extra chewing means more saliva is produced. Saliva is, you will recall, alkaline. The increased flow of this alkaline fluid into the stomach helps lower stomach acidity and, thus, reduces the risk of irritation to the mucous membranes there. Whether or not this theory is true, a high-fibre diet has many other benefits with regard to problems with digestion and so is worth adopting anyway.

Continuously high alcohol intakes seem to cause more duodenal ulcers than gastric ones and so should be avoided wherever possible.

Tea and coffee should also be kept to a minimum so as to avoid encouraging extra acid to be secreted in the stomach.

To avoid developing or to recover from duodenal ulcers, you should follow a low-fat diet. Some fats are necessary as they contain vitamins A, D and E and EFAs. The ones that provide such nutrients are the vegetable and fish oils. Saturated animal fats – found in fatty cuts of meat, the skin of poultry, butter, full-cream dairy products and in manufactured products like pies, pastries, cakes, biscuits and so on – need to be cut right back, and the fats which are eaten need to come from vegetable oils, nuts and seeds and oily fish.

There could be a need for EFAs to be taken as supplements. It has been found that men suffering from duodenal ulcers have significantly lower amounts of the EFA linoleic acid in their abdominal walls than do healthy men. As the amount of linoleic acid storedin fat in the body reflects the amount that is eaten, it wouldseem that duodenal ulcer sufferers have a lower intake than non- sufferers. As mentioned under Gastric Ulcers, in Chapter 4, the linings of the mucous membranes may be protected by prosta-glandins, substances made from linoleic acid. A good supple-mentary source of EFAs that the body can easily turn into prostaglandins is evening primrose oil.

Gallbladder Problems

When the gallbladder starts producing gallstones, eating can become a complete misery. Soon after indulging in a fatty meal or even just a fatty snack, a person with gallstones can experience severe flatu-lence along with gripping chest pains. So, what is the gallbladder and why does it cause symptoms of indigestion when it goes wrong?

The gallbladder sits alongside the intestine. It is a thin-walled, small, green, muscular sack or bag that, like a miniature version of the stomach, can expand and contract in size depending on the volume of its contents. It is around 10 cm (4 in) long and can hold between 30 and 50 ml (1 and 2 fl oz), which is about a third of a small yogurt pot. The gallbladder looks a bit like a two-tentacled octopus, with its rounded 'head' connected to both the liver and the top part of the small intestine by two different ducts or tubes.

The gallbladder's function is to store a thick, liquid substance called bile and to release it into the intestine when required. The liver makes the bile and sends it to the gallbladder via one of the ducts. It stays in the gallbladder until the hormone called CCK arrives on the scene, instructing it to shoot bile into the other duct, which leads into the intestine. CCK also has the effect of relaxing the valve located where the duct joins the intestine, thus allowing the bile in.

Bile has one main constituent that helps indigestion – bile salts. Bile salts help break down and emulsify fats in the intestine and distribute them evenly throughout the rest of the chyme.

As mentioned earlier, this is a bit like what happens when milk is homogenized, when the creamy part is thoroughly mixed in with the watery part of the milk, making the fat and water homogenous.

The bile salts, therefore, physically separate the big globules of fat – eaten, for example, in the form of cheese, butter, margarine or ice-cream – breaking them down into millions of tiny fatty droplets.

Bile also contains, among other things, cholesterol and pigments. It is the pigment that gives our stools their character-istic colour. Without bile, they would look a grey white colour and also contain fatty streaks as, without bile, fats are not properly digested or absorbed into the body.

The hormone CCK, which, you remember, stimulates the gall-bladder to release bile, is itself released when the contents of the stomach moving into the intestine are rich in fats.

Problems with the gallbladder occur when it makes gallstones from cholesterol. Bile salts normally keep levels of cholesterol at the correct level, but if there is too much cholesterol for the bile salts to deal with, then the cholesterol crystallizes, forming the so-called 'stones'. These sit in the gallbladder itself and/or in the duct, obstructing the flow of bile. When the gallbladder or duct contracts in response to a fatty meal, the sharp crystals dig into the walls and cause agonizing pain, which spreads throughout the right side of the chest region, causing severeindigestion.

Gallstones are known to be a complication associated with obesity. It is well worth shedding excess weight to help avoid developing them. Also, people who are overweight experience worse symptoms when they have gallstones than do their normal weight counterparts. In the late 1980s, 88,837 women aged between 34 and 59 years were selected for a study and followed up over a 4-year period. They completed detailed food and alcohol intake diaries and their weights were recorded. It was found that there was a link between diet and weight in that the more overweight the women, the more likely they were to develop gall-stones. One woman who was 41 and over 25 kg (about 4 stone/ 56 lb) overweight went on a 1,000 calories a day diet. Over 15 months, she lost 19 kg (3 stone/42 lb), during which period her gallstones disappeared. After 19 months, she was down to her ideal weight and her gallbladder was working properly.

It would seem sensible, judging from the picture you can build from this research, that getting down to or keeping to a normal bodyweight is a must to give your gallbladder a chance of working properly.

Gallstones can be surgically removed. It is also possible to dissolve the crystals. Nowadays, however, they are more likely to be treated by ultrasound vibrations, which pulverize, or lasers, which vaporize them.

Dietary Advice

A low-fat diet is often prescribed for people who suffer from gall-stones. Its effectiveness has not been completely tried and tested with enough clinical studies to know for certain whether or not it is truly effective. However, it does seem to make sense that if fatty foods stimulate the gallbladder to contract and deliver bile to the intestine, that a low-fat diet will reduce its activity and, thus, discomfort. Very often, it's a case of trial and error when working out just how much fat can be tolerated by an individual, and it is worth experimenting with.

Most people in the West eat diets with around 40 to 45 per cent of the total calories coming from fat. This needs to be reduced to 35 per cent for normal fit people. If you suffer from gallstones, you could try reducing your fat intake to more like the 30 per cent level to see if this helps improve symptoms. For a woman who eats about 2,000 calories a day, 30 per cent of this would be 600 calories. As 1 g of fat contains 9 calories, this would mean that she would need to keep the total grams of fat eaten in a day down to around 67 g (2½ oz). For a man eating a total of 2,550 calories a day, 30 per cent of this would be 765. This would translate into a daily total of 85 g (3½ oz) of fat.

For most people, meat and meat products, like sausages, beef-burgers, meat pies and pasties, the spreading fats, like butter and margarine, cooking oils, full-fat milk and dairy products, such as cheeses, cream and full-fat yogurts, are the main sources of fat in the diet because they are eaten on a daily basis. Fats hidden within other foods, like savoury snacks, pastries, biscuits, cakes and puddings and other desserts, also add a considerable and increasing amount of fat to the diet and need to be carefully controlled when on a low-fat diet.

Over the last few years, there has been an enormous growth in the number of reduced and low-fat products appearing on the supermarket shelves, and these can help enormously when you are following a low-fat plan.

Skimmed milk is now readily available, as are reduced or virtually fat-free dairy products, including yogurts, fromage frais, cheeses, ready-made custards and milk puddings. There are also many low-fat and very low-fat spreads, although if you don't like any of them, just use the minimum amount of butter or a traditional margarine. Low-fat ready meals fill the freezer and chill cabinets, and all kinds of reduced-fat crisps, chips, sausages, burgers, dressings and even ice-creams are now on the market.

The following lists of foods – divided into very low-fat, low-fat, medium- and high- fat categories – can help guide you as to the good and bad foods. However, check before you buy because some reduced-fat products are still, compared to other foods, relatively quite fatty. Reduced-fat Cheddar, for example, is still a medium-fat food.

Very Low-fat Foods (less than 5 g per 100 g/⅛ oz per 4 oz)

- skimmed milk
- low-fat yogurt
- egg white
- cottage cheese
- turkey breast, skinless, grilled
- white fish, poached or steamed
- shellfish, steamed
- all vegetables, including potatoes, cooked without fat
- salad vegetables, without dressing
- beans, peas and lentils
- plain boiled sweets

- jam and honey
- sauces and pickles
- Marmite (yeast extract)
- bread
- pasta
- breakfast cereals
- crispbreads
- meringues
- jellies
- custard and rice pudding, made with skimmed milk
- fruits, fresh, frozen, canned

Low-fat Foods (5–10 g fat per 100 g/⅛–¼ oz per 4 oz)

- ham
- lean steak, grilled
- lean roast beef, leg pork, leg lamb, roast chicken, without skin
- kidneys, grilled
- pilchards
- roast potatoes
- oven chips
- cream and thick soups
- muesli (granola)
- Ready Brek
- soft rolls
- currant buns
- sponge, such as Swiss roll
- trifle
- ice-cream
- apple crumble

Medium-fat Foods
(containing 10–20 g fat per 100 g/¼–¾ oz per 4 oz)

- full-fat yogurt
- boiled eggs

- Feta cheese
- curd cheese
- reduced-fat Cheddar
- lean back bacon, grilled
- rump steak, fried
- mince, stewed
- lean lamb and pork chops
- chicken, roasted, with skin
- beefburgers, hamburgers
- livers, fried
- cod in batter, fried
- salmon, tinned
- sardines
- fish fingers
- scampi, fried
- thick-cut chips/french fries
- olives
- Mars bar
- toffees
- cream crackers
- rich tea biscuits
- oatcakes
- ginger nuts
- wafers
- rock and madeira cakes
- doughnuts
- scones
- fruit cakes
- pancakes
- sponge pudding
- fruit pies
- lemon meringue pie

High-fat Foods
(containing more than 20 g fat per 100 g/¾ oz per 4 oz)

- butter
- margarine
- cream, all types
- oils, all types
- mayonnaise, including low-fat varieties
- low-fat spreads
- salad cream, including low-fat varieties
- peanut butter
- eggs, scrambled and fried
- Scotch eggs
- Stilton
- cream cheeses
- Cheddar, Cheshire
- Parmesan
- Edam
- cheese spreads
- quiche
- Welsh rarebit
- streaky bacon, fried
- lamb and pork chops, with fat
- roast duck, with skin and fat
- liver pâté
- luncheon meat
- pork sausages
- sausage rolls
- pork pies
- pasties and meat pies
- taramasalata
- whitebait, fried
- chips (french fries), deep-fried
- crisps (potato chips), normal and low-fat varieties
- avocados
- soya beans

- nuts
- milk chocolate
- chocolate biscuits
- filled wafers
- custard creams
- shortbread
- pastry, all types
- Victoria sponge cake
- cream cakes
- pies
- cheesecakes

As to other pieces of advice, interestingly it has also been shown that women who skipped breakfast or only had coffee at the start of the day had a greater incidence of gallstones than did those who ate breakfast. So, taking breakfast may help prevent gallstones occurring.

In addition, it has been suggested and observed that frequent consumption of smoked foods also seems to encourage the formation of gallstones. Commonly consumed smoked foods include bacon and smoked mackerel.

The good news, though, is that a moderate intake of alcohol may actually help to reduce the incidence of gallstones.

Cholesterol in the Diet

It is commonly thought that when foods known to be rich in cholesterol, such as egg yolks, fish roe and shellfish are eaten, the cholesterol levels in the blood will rise once the foods have been digested. In fact, scientists have never been able to show that blood cholesterol rises after eating such foods. Most of the cholesterol in the blood is made by the body itself. Levels of cholesterol rise if the diet is rich in saturated fats, found in animal fats, dairy products, coconut oil and coconut cream and foods containing these fats.

The incidence of gallstones in France, India, Japan, Portugal, South Africa, Sweden and Uganda was studied back in 1978 and the results showed that in those countries where total calories and fat intakes were lower and vegetable intakes higher, few people had gallstones. After the Second World War, the incidence of gallstones increased in France over a 20-year period. The increases occurred as the diets increased in total calories and fats.

Studies that compared vegetarian women with non-vegetarian women have revealed that, as a group, vegetarian women have less than half the incidence of gallstones of their meat-eating sisters. The researchers carrying out the study believed that this finding could be attributed to the fact that the vegetarians ate less fat and more fibre.

From this it is clear that to help reduce cholesterol levels in the body, it is necessary to keep consumption of saturated fats well down. Eating foods rich in so-called 'soluble fibre' found in, for example, pulses, apples and oats, helps keep cholesterol levels down too.

Nausea

Most of us assume that nausea starts in the stomach. While this can happen, queasy feelings often in fact start in the duodenum due to local disturbances to its lining such as inflammation or ulceration. Messages are sent from the nerves in this upper part of the small intestine to the brain, which in turn feeds them back to the stomach. The distressing sensation it creates often leads to vomiting. Vomiting unsettles the peace of the tract, making the throat sore and leaving the mouth very acidic. It is important to try to calm the system by taking some rest and trying to drink some water to keep your fluid levels up.

Food Intolerances

Some people are born with and others develop intolerances to certain foods. These are not allergic reactions which involve the immune system, but are reproducible, unpleasant, non-psychological reactions to a specific food or food ingredient. It seems that the small intestine is particularly vulnerable to certain of these which, if not corrected, can cause symptoms which range from the uncomfortable to the potentially life threatening. For a calm and cleansed digestive tract, intolerances need to be diagnosed nearest the time of their onset as possible so that offending foods can be removed and order restored as quickly as possible.

Lactose Intolerance

Lactose is the sugar found in milk. It is known as a disaccharide or double sugar because it consists of the two single sugars glucose and galactose which are joined together. Lactose cannot be absorbed across the intestinal wall and into the blood until it has been broken down into glucose and galactose by the enzyme lactase, which sits in the wall.

A lack of the enzyme lactase gives rise to lactose intolerance – that is, the inability to break down lactose. This means the lactose passes undigested from the small intestine into the large intestine. Bacteria in the large intestine start fermenting the lactose, producing gases and irritating acids. These by-products of lactose fermentation lead to bloating, abdominal cramps and terrible wind. It is believed that just 2 g (⅛ oz) of lactose can lead to the production of 1,400 ml (50 fl oz) of hydrogen gas. One lactose-intolerant man was once recorded to have passed wind 141 times after consuming two pints of milk, a feat which made it into the *Guinness Book of Records*. The presence of lactose in the large intestine also has the effect of pulling in water and sugar from the surrounding blood vessels, which leads to profuse diarrhoea.

Lactose intolerance is usually an inherited problem. All new-born babies have enough lactase to cope with lactose in breastmilk or that found in infant formulas. After weaning, however, lactase activity decreases in all mammals, including humans. Lactase levels usually drop between the ages of two and five, and drop further in some than others. A child may start having symptoms of intolerance as late as when they first go to school.

In many parts of the world, entire races have very low levels of the lactase enzyme and thus cannot tolerate milk and dairy products. Many Asians, Native Americans and Japanese are in this position. Lactose intolerance can also start in later life, developing, for example, following intestinal infections, gastric surgery or a course of antibiotics or anti-inflammatory medication.

Usually the intolerance to milk's sugar is not absolute, meaning that the child or adult can cope with small amounts of dairy foods on a daily basis. Cheese and yogurt do not have high concentrations of lactose and are sometimes better tolerated as, fortunately, is chocolate.

Once diagnosed by your doctor, it is advisable to see a dietitian and work out a lactose-free diet for a specific period of time. Gradually, under his or her guidance, it is possible to reintroduce some milk products to assess how much, if any, can be tolerated. Since dairy products are such a valuable source of calcium, especially for the growing child, it is crucial that other sources of this essential mineral are consumed on a regular basis to ensure optimum bone mass is achieved and maintained. This requires a degree of dedication to the cause, but is well worth it for future health. Today it is also possible to buy calcium-enriched soya milk which is a very useful alternative.

Calcium-rich Foods

Foods	Mg of calcium per 100 g (4 oz) of food
Tahini	680
Sesame seeds	670
Tofu	510
Spinach	170
Sunflower seeds	110
Ready-to-eat apricots	73
Kidney beans	71
Peanuts	60
Peanut butter	37

Some people are intolerant to the proteins in milk and not the lactose. They would need to avoid the following foods:

all foods containing milk, cheese, butter, margarine, cream,
cheese, yogurt, skimmed milk powder, non-fat milk solids,
caseinates, whey, lactalbumin and lactose
biscuits (cookies)
breads, buns and bread mixes
breakfast cereals
cakes and cake mixes
flavoured crisps (potato chips)
gravy mixes
malted drinks
puddings and mixes, ice cream, custard, instant whips
sauces and cream soups
sausages and batters
sweets such as chocolate, fudge, toffee.

A full and comprehensive list of lactose- and milk protein-free foods
is available from your local registered dietitian. Recognizing and
dealing with milk intolerances is crucial to the settled functioning
of the digestive system.

Gluten Intolerance

Coeliac disease is the condition which arises when an individual's
small intestine lining is damaged by gluten, the protein found in
wheat and rye, and by similar proteins found in barley and possibly
oats. The long finger-like projections called villi which make up the
wall of the small intestine become flattened when a person is intolerant to gluten, which means the surface area of this part of the
digestive system is drastically reduced. This in turn leads to food
speeding through without having a chance to be broken down and
absorbed. Weight loss inevitably follows and the stools become
either large, pale and with an offensive smell, or become loose, later
developing into diarrhoea. Vomiting may also occur.

In children, a normal baby who is weaned onto foods containing
gluten will start by refusing foods and then begin to lose weight. The
child will become listless, and the stools change as described. The
abdomen will swell, developing into what appears to be a pot belly.

In adults, the classic symptoms of indigestion can be the first signs of gluten intolerance. These could be anything from abdominal fullness and discomfort in the stomach region to diarrhoea, pain, vomiting and terrible tiredness. The changes to the stools may be a tell-tale sign, as they become pale, bulky and dreadfully smelly due to fat not being absorbed by the flattened intestinal walls and therefore remaining in the faeces.

Around one person in 1,850 is believed to have this intolerance to gluten in the UK, and although it runs in families the disease is not actually inherited. Quite what causes a person to become gluten-intolerant is still not really understood. Explanations have ranged from the gluten being intrinsically toxic to certain people because they lack a detoxifying enzyme, to the disease being an allergic reaction by the gut wall to the gluten. Neither theory really explains why it strikes a wide range of ages, or why different symptoms are experienced by different people.

Diagnosis, however, is crucial if digestive health is to be restored. This can only be done by a specialist doctor who takes a sample of the small intestine and studies it under the microscope to see if the villi are flattened.

Treatment for coeliac disease is to avoid gluten in the diet as much as possible. There are two main sources. The obvious sources are foods made from wheat flour or which contain barley or oats – bread, cereals, cakes, biscuits, pies and pastries, for example. Second, there are the less obvious sources. These are manufactured or processed foods that contain any of these cereals as fillers, thickeners, for bulking up and so on. They may be in the form of gluten, wheat starch, rusk or hydrolysed vegetable protein of wheat origin. They are added to the most unlikely things, such as sweets, as well as slightly more obvious ones, such as white sauces in boil-in-the-bag cod in parsley sauce and tinned foods like chicken in sauce.

Gluten-containing foods to avoid	Gluten-free alternatives
Cereals and cereal products	
Wheat, wholemeal, wholewheat and wheatmeal flours. Bran, barley, rye, rye flour, pasta and semolina.	Arrowroot, buckwheat, corn cornflour, maize and maize flour. Gluten-free flour, potato flour, rice and rice flour. Sago, soya and soya flour. Tapioca.
Cereals made from wheat, barley or rye, such as muesli, Shredded Wheat, Sugar Puffs and Weetabix.	Rice Krispies and cornflakes.
Baked products made from wheat, barley, rye flour, suet and semolina.	Gluten-free baked biscuits, (cookies) bread, cakes and gluten-free pasta.
Crispbreads and starch-reduced bread and rolls. Ice-cream wafers and cones, plus Communion wafers.	
Milk and milk products	
Artificial cream containing flour. Yogurt containing muesli/granola.	Fresh, dried, condensed, evaporated, skimmed, sterilized. Fresh or tinned cream. Most yogurts.
Cheese spreads containing flour, which many do – check the labels.	Cheddar, curd and cream cheeses.
Egg dishes	
Eggs cooked with flour, such as Scotch eggs, eggs with white sauces. Quiches and egg flans.	Cooked without breadcrumbs and sauces.
Fats and oils	
Suet contains flour.	All butters, margarines, oils, lard and dripping.

Meat and fish

Savoury pies and puddings made with flour. Any meat or fish with stuffings, breadcrumbs or suet. Sausages and burgers with bread-crumbs or rusk (check the packaging). Battered and crumbed fish, like fish fingers and fishcakes.

Plain meat and fish.
Plain tinned fish. Check packaging of burgers and pre-packed meat – some are gluten-free.

Vegetables, fruits and nuts

Tinned vegetables in sauces, such as creamed mushrooms. Potato croquettes. TVP containing wheat.

Fresh, tinned, cooked, dried and frozen, pulses and soya. Some baked beans – check the labels.

Fruit in fruit pies, crumbles and cakes.

Fresh, cooked, tinned, dried and frozen.

Nuts in cooked products and crackers and dry-roasted nuts.

Fresh, plain, salted.

Jams, sweets and desserts

Sweets containing or rolled in flour. Smarties, marshmallows, liquorice and Twix.

Sugar, glucose, jam, honey, marmalade, treacle, molasses, some mincemeat – check the label. Plain ice lollies/pops.

Puddings and desserts with flour, breadcrumbs and suet, such as pies crumbles and summer puddings. Ice-cream cones and wafers.

Jellies and milk puddings made from permitted cereals.
Check the labels of ice-cream and instant desserts as some are gluten-free. Not semolina.

Drinks

Barley-based instant coffee, barley-flavoured drinks. Bengers, malted

Tea, pure, instant or fresh ground coffee, cocoa, fizzy

drinks, such as Horlicks. Home-brewed beer, cloudy real ale and hot drinks from vending machines.

drinks, squashes and cordials, fresh fruit juices, wines, spirits, beer and lagers.

Soups, sauces and seasonings

Soups thickened with the cereals wheat, barley, rye or pasta. Bisto.

Home-made soups with suitable thickeners. Certain brands of tinned and dried soups. Certain gravy brownings. Check the packaging.

Some peppers, ready-mixed spices and curry powders.

Fresh peppers and herbs. Check the labels on other seasonings, mustards and powders.

Note: Beware that some medicines contain gluten, so check with the pharmacist or your doctor before taking anything if you are unsure.

Wheat Intolerance

In some cases, people are sensitive to wheat and wheat-containing foods, but when tested for coeliac disease are clearly not intolerant to gluten. While they must avoid wheat and wheat-containing foods, they are able to eat oats and barley. People sensitive to wheat are often those who eat a lot of it in breakfast cereals, pasta and bread. Wheat and other cereal staple crops were only introduced into our diets around 10,000 years ago (a blink of an eye in evolutionary terms), and it is believed that is why the problem is so common. Many people have not evolved the necessary digestive equipment to deal with the increasingly large quantities we throw at it on a daily basis.

With the help of a dietitian, the following foods need to be eliminated on a wheat-free diet:

some drinking chocolates and Horlicks
biscuits/cookies
cakes
bread – all types
breakfast cereals made from wheat
some cheese spreads, processed cheese and packet suet
some tinned fish and fish paste plus fish cooked in batter,
breadcrumbs or a sauce
flours and cereals including wheatgerm, semolina, pasta and
noodles
some canned meats and many ready meals, pies, sausage rolls,
meat paste, paté and sausages
pastry
puddings (check the labels)
soups.

In addition, always check labels for the words 'wheat starch', 'edible'
or 'modified starch', 'cereal filler', 'bran', 'rusk', 'cereal binder' or
'cereal protein'.

Fructose Intolerance

Rather like lactose intolerance, some people cannot cope with the
fruit sugar fructose. Fructose is a single sugar found in fruits, and
attached to glucose in table sugar. Thus all fruits and foods
containing ordinary sugar need to be avoided. Fortunately, children
born with fructose intolerance soon develop an innate and strong
dislike of anything sweet-tasting, so they remain well as long as they
are not forced to eat such foods. Since fruit and fruit juices must be
avoided, it is important to ensure children get plenty of vegetables
which supply the body with vitamin C, such as red, green, yellow
and orange peppers, potatoes, sweet potatoes and, if you can
persuade them, dark green leafy vegetables like spinach, broccoli
and cabbage.

— 6 —
The Large Intestine

This section of the digestive tract is called 'large' because of its diameter rather than its length. It is half a metre (1½ feet) shorter than the small intestine and considerably fatter. Two main functions of the large intestine are to absorb water from indigestible food residues and to eliminate them from the body as semi-solid faeces.

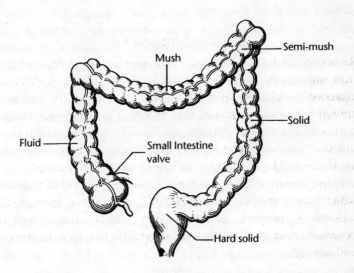

The semi-fluid contents of the small intestine are gradually turned into solids in the large intestine.

The large intestine is divided into five sections:

1. caecum
2. appendix
3. colon
4. rectum
5. anal canal.

Most of the main nutrients from food and drink have been absorbed once they reach the large intestine, so there is no reason to have all the little villi found on the surface of the small intestine. The surface is therefore flatter.

Although it is not having to secrete enzymes to break down nutrients like the small intestine, it would be wrong to give the impression that the large intestine is just a waste-processing plant. There are many, many metabolic processes taking place here which influence the health of the overall digestive system.

For example it actually synthesizes vitamin K, which is then absorbed across the large intestine's lining into the bloodstream. This role is vital since most of us eat insufficient vitamin K in our diets and it is crucial for the mechanisms involved in blood-clotting as well as energy metabolism. The large intestine is also capable of making the vitamins B_{12}, B_1 and B_2.

In addition to synthesizing certain vitamins, the large intestine converts sugars and starches which have not been absorbed by the small intestine into so-called short-chain fatty acids, which then cross over into the bloodstream and can be used by the body as a source of energy (or calories). In herbivores this short-chain fatty acid production provides a significant proportion of their calories, up to 22 per cent. In humans it is much smaller but still important.

The large intestine is also very much involved with water balance in the body. It receives large amounts of water from the small intestine, and an astonishing 7 litres ($1^1/2$ gallons) can be absorbed from it by the bloodstream in just 24 hours.

The large intestine is also home to millions and millions of bacteria and yeast, known as the gut flora. The flora feed on the remains of our meals, and on the whole are harmless. In fact, many are essential to the well-being of the gut. In a healthy person the gut flora get along just fine and create a balanced community. They literally cover the whole surface of the colon, many helping to prevent disease-causing bacteria from invading and taking over.

At certain times this finely balanced ecosystem may be disturbed, for example during a bout of food poisoning or through long-term use of antibiotics. Abnormalities in gut flora have been discovered in people suffering from Irritable Bowel Syndrome (see page 54), *Candida* overgrowth (see page 61) and similar diseases.

The large intestine does not move anything like as quickly as the small intestine and stomach. In fact, it can be rather like a lazy lizard basking in the sun, making the odd slow shuffling movement every half hour or so. By means of such movements, the residues of digestion are gradually shoved on round the colon until they reach the rectum. At this point nerves tell the rectum to contract and the valve to the anal canal opens. Once faeces enter the rectum, messages are sent to the brain and we then consciously decide whether or not to open the final valve of the whole system, the external anal valve, to allow expulsion of the stools.

The contents of the faeces, the exact components of the gut flora and the speed at which waste moves through the large intestine can all be significantly influenced by the food we eat. The overall health of this part of the digestive system is also intimately connected to our emotional well-being. Most of us will have experienced 'intestinal hurry' due to stress or fear at some time in our lives. Cleansing of the large intestine is possible through careful dietary choices and a thoughtful long-term approach to choices of foods and drinks.

Dietary Advice

As a rule, a bulky diet – in other words, a high-fibre diet – can, surprisingly, often be of help at such times. Instead of aggravating the system and rushing gut contents through at even greater speed, it can help bind the stools up a bit, making them bulkier and therefore slowing them down.

Irritable Bowel Syndrome

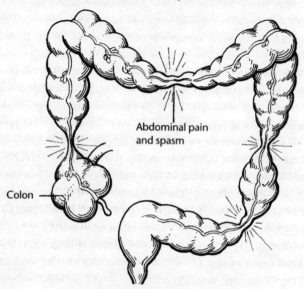

Abdominal pain
and spasm

Colon

The large intestine of an IBS sufferer.

IBS has been identified as being related, in some women, to the pre-menstrual time of the month, and it is also often said to be brought on by stress, major surgery such as a hysterectomy, or the long-term use of antibiotics.

The one common link between all IBS sufferers, though, is that no physical ailment, such as Crohn's disease, ulcerative colitis, diverticulitis or cancer, can be identified. A great deal of specialist hospital time and equipment is necessary to eliminate all these other possible causes of the symptoms. Only after all the examinations have been carried out on the gut, and no such underlying cause can be detected, can a true diagnosis of IBS be made.

Defining what is normal for the bowels has always been a moot point. Some people can pass stools twice a day and think it is normal, while others could go three days and not consider themselves to be constipated. Some may always feel bloated after eating and consider it to be just a side-effect of eating and drinking, while others may find it uncomfortable enough to seek help. The incidence of IBS symptoms could in fact be even higher than the figures currently quoted as some sufferers may well never seek help or advice.

IBS is not a single entity and can be linked to many situations. Stress from, for example, divorce, moving house, losing a job or the death of someone close, hyperventilation, musculoskeletal problems and hormonal imbalances have all been cited as causes. That there are so many potential causes means that there is not one single effective treatment. Some doctors prescribe antispasmodic drugs, others bulking agents and some even tranquillizers. Dietary advice can also be helpful to some sufferers.

IBS provides yet another example of just how intimately the gut's reactions and the emotions can be linked. Taking time out for yourself to enjoy relaxation such as swimming, sitting in a sauna or steam room, having a massage, going to yoga or Pilates classes or simply taking a peaceful walk should all be considered alongside any dietary modifications you might consider.

Dietary Advice

Those who have specific symptoms of abdominal distension and wind may find that cutting out vegetables of the brassica family, such as cabbage, Brussels sprouts and broccoli, and pulses, such as red kidney, baked and black-eyed beans, as well as lentils, peas and chickpeas, and apples, grapes and raisins may help.

In the past, high-fibre diets have been recommended for IBS sufferers. Additions of up to 7 g (about ⅛ oz) a day of wheat bran has, for example, been suggested for people who are suffering constipation as a result of IBS. Today, however, there is a movement away from bran, in recognition of the fact that intolerances to certain foods could be more to blame.

In order to detect which foods may be causing a specific person's problems, an exclusion diet needs to be followed. Research has proven that this has been effective in treating between 48 and 67 per cent of IBS patients. The exclusion diet developed in Cambridge at

Addenbrookes Hospital is based on the plan set out below, but note that any kind of exclusion diet should only be undertaken with the permission of your GP and the guidance of a dietitian. This is necessary because it is not just a case of leaving out certain foods. It has to be done in a structured way and one that will provide meaningful results. The diet followed during the exclusion period and any diet prescribed afterwards for maintenance must be nutritionally adequate for the person concerned and this needs to be worked out with a qualified dietician.

Foods	Not Allowed	Allowed
Meat	Preserved meats, bacon, sausages	All other meats
Fish	Smoked fish, shellfish	White fish
Vegetables	Potatoes, onions, sweetcorn	All other vegetables
Fruit	Citrus fruits	All other fruit
Cereals	Wheat, barley, oats, corn, rye	Rice, tapioca, millet, buckwheat
Oils	Corn oil, vegetable oil	Sunflower, soya, safflower, olive oils
Dairy	Cows' and goat's milk, butter margarines, yogurts, cheese, eggs	Soya milk, milk-free margarine
Beverages	Tea, coffee, fruit squashes, grapefruit juice, alcohol, tap water	Herbal teas, apple, pineapple, tomato juices, mineral water
Other	Chocolate, yeast, vinegar, preservatives	Carob, salt, herbs, spices, sugar, honey

This is followed for two weeks and then the symptoms are reassessed. This needs to be done by your doctor. If there has been no improvement, then the person will be advised to return to their normal diet. If symptoms have cleared, however, the foods that were excluded are reintroduced, one at a time at two-day intervals in the following order:

- tap water
- potatoes
- cows' milk
- yeast
- tea
- rye
- butter
- onions
- eggs
- oats
- coffee
- chocolate
- barley
- citrus fruits
- corn
- cheese
- white wine
- shellfish
- yogurt
- vinegar
- wheat
- nuts
- preservatives.

When following such a plan, you need to keep a really close check on your symptoms and write them down on a daily basis.

Just to reinforce the point made above, though, it is vital that this kind of food exclusion diet is followed under the supervision of your doctor and a dietitian, who can ensure that the diet is kept to and that the food eaten is sufficiently rich in nutrients for your personal requirements to avoid any adverse effects of the exclusion.

After the results of the exclusion period and reintroduction of foods are known, how you should mix the foods that have been found to be well tolerated will also need to be worked out with your health-care provider to make sure that your diet will be providing all the necessary nutrients to maintain good health. It's no good having a diet that relieves the symptoms of IBS but is deficient in essential vitamins or minerals as such deficiencies will manifest themselves as problems in the future, such as anaemia from iron deficiency or osteoporosis (brittle bones) due to a lack of calcium.

Research, again carried out in Cambridge, showed that the following foods created symptoms of intolerance in the following percentages of patients:

- wheat, 60 per cent
- corn, 44 per cent
- milk, 44 per cent
- cheese, 39 per cent
- oats, 34 per cent
- coffee, 33 per cent
- rye, 30 per cent
- eggs, 26 per cent
- butter, 25 per cent
- tea, 25 per cent
- citrus, 24 per cent
- barley, 24 per cent
- yogurt, 24 per cent
- chocolate, 22 per cent
- nuts, 22 per cent
- onions, 22 per cent
- potatoes, 20 per cent
- preservatives, 20 per cent.

Probiotics and IBS

Researchers in Sweden have discovered that altering the gut flora by introducing probiotics ('good' bacteria) can significantly decrease the amount of pain and flatulence suffered in patients with IBS. To date the study of the influence of gut flora in people with IBS has not received much attention. The Swedish scientists recognized, however, that because some bacterial strains are more prone to gas production than others, if these can be reduced some relief of symptoms may be possible.

To test their theory, patients were given a fruit juice to drink which had been fortified with a member of the *Lactobacillus* family, a group of bacteria which are normally found in the healthy colon. By the end of the experiments, the scientists had been proven right. Adding *Lactobacillus plantarum* to the IBS sufferer's diet via the fruit juice had the effect of knocking out many of the gas-producing bacteria.

Flatulence decreased by half in 44 per cent of the group who had the drink with added probiotics. They also reported improved bowel movements. The drink is available in the UK under the name Proviva and can be found in good supermarkets.

'Alternative Testing'

It is possible to have a wide range of tests done that claim to prove food intolerances for IBS and other problems. Vega machines, hair analysis, cytotoxic tests – the list goes on. None has any scientific justification. Immunological abnormalities occur in some patients with known food intolerances. These can be detected by means of special tests, but they are notoriously tricky to do and can be unreliable.

Some scientists believe that food intolerances can develop due to a change in the flora in bowels due to antibiotic treatment in the past. Changes in flora have indeed been found in IBS patients who identify an aggravating food, remove it from the diet and then reintroduce it. Testing stools for changes in flora to detect food intolerances is not yet a recognized technique and it remains to be seen whether it could become so in the future.

The only reliable dietary treatment method available at the moment is that of following a proper exclusion diet under medical and dietetic supervision, such as the one suggested above.

Bloating

Bloating may be due to a food intolerance. Common intolerances that lead to bloating include an inability to deal with the milk sugar, lactose (for further details, see page 43).

Bloating can, however, be explained as being an occasional reaction to a certain type of food, such as cabbage or swede, or the result of an excessive amount of wind accumulating in the intestine. A sudden influx of high-fibre foods, especially pulses, can have this effect, too, while swallowing too much air is another cause. This last explanation may sound rather strange, but we all swallow air every time we speak, eat and drink. Eating in a rush, having large quantities of foods containing air, such as soufflés and meringues, and gulping down lots of carbonated drinks, all these things encourage extra air to be swallowed. However, this is easily remedied.

Dietary Advice

Again, the way in which you approach eating and drinking affects your digestion. Taking time and sitting down are essential. Chewing thoroughly and taking the whole process slowly will help reduce the amount of air swallowed with food. Gulping down foods and drinks will mean that you are taking in quite large quantities of air with each mouthful. Talking while eating has a similar effect, as does eating with your mouth open.

Avoid carbonated drinks. These introduce more unwanted air. Use plain water and still juices rather than fizzy water and orange, lemon, cola and other such drinks. It helps, too, to drink from a glass rather than straight from a bottle or can.

Chewing gum also causes you to swallow extra air. If you are having problems with excess wind, then try avoiding gum for a while to see if things improve at all.

When increasing the fibre content of your diet, remember to do so gradually. Start by making small, single changes, for example, just swapping from white to wholemeal bread. Gradually progress to including extra fruit and vegetables and, finally, start increasing the amounts of pulses, like beans and peas, in your diet. This allows the intestine time to get used to these foods and to produce the correct bacteria in the large intestine to deal with them, which will help keep the problem of bloating – which often accompanies a switch to a high-fibre diet – under control.

If bloating is a symptom of irritable bowel syndrome (IBS), see the previous section.

Candida

Candida albicans is one of the yeasts that we all have growing and living in our gut, and in women it is also found in the vagina. While most problems with overgrowth of *Candida* occur in the vagina, where it causes thrush, it can also affect the urinary tract and bladder, the throat, where it causes soreness, the mouth, leading to yellow patches and, when the immune system is under a lot of pressure, can affect other organs such as the eyes and liver. It also seems to affect the digestive system, causing bloating, pains and cramps, diarrhoea or IBS.

While *Candida* lives naturally in the gut, the strange thing is that those with a *Candida* problem don't appear to have any more of this yeast than those who don't suffer any adverse symptoms. Possibly they just become more sensitive to normal levels. The important thing to note is that, whatever the reason, once patients try a low-sugar, low-yeast diet, symptoms of thrush often seem to disappear along with the intestinal symptoms of diarr-hoea and wind. Your doctor can refer you to a dietitian who will advise you how to follow an appropriate diet.

Some trials have been carried out, with interesting results. One experiment, for example, showed that *Candida albicans* fails to grow in human saliva unless it is supplemented with glucose.

A trial was carried out in 1984 in which 100 women who had recurring *Candida* infections of the vagina had the sugar in their urine measured. When sugar appeared in the urine, it related to a time of excessive sugar intake. When sugar was eliminated as much as possible, there was a dramatic reduction in the incidence and severity of the *Candida* infections.

In an experimental study back in 1966, of 255 patients with long-term urticaria, 49 of them reacted to *Candida albicans* antigens, and 55 per cent of them also reacted to brewer's yeast. After treatment with a low-yeast diet and anti-fungal therapy, 27 out of the 49 experienced a clinical cure.

It has been suggested that a diet which excludes simple carbohydrate and yeast-rich foods will prevent candidiasis by depriving the organisms of a suitable environment in which to grow. This kind of diet requires the person involved to avoid foods containing simple sugars, which means no adding of sugar to foods or drinks at the table or eating foods rich in it, such as sweets, cakes, ice-creams and desserts, fruit juices, condiments and tinned fruits in syrup. It also involves cutting out yeast-containing foods and drinks, such as malted products, mushrooms, cheeses, peanuts and alcoholic drinks, as well as vinegar-containing foods and vitamin and mineral tablets, unless they are sugar- and yeast-free, and antibiotics.

The debate continues, but there are some respected clinics in which doctors and dietitians working together have seen improvements in patients who follow such diets and take the drug nystatin (prescribed for fungal infections).

Piles

Piles are largely believed to be related to over straining when trying to go to the loo. The best advice is to try to follow a high fibre diet and take plenty of fluids.

7
Cleansing the System of Poisons

Every day the digestive system is presented with 'foreign substances', such as bacteria and natural and chemical toxins, and it generally deals with these effectively and safely, killing them off, detoxifying them or simply coping with their presence. Sometimes, however, a food or drink may contain too much of a particular infectious or toxic agent, or be harbouring one against which the body has no defences.

When things get out of balance and poisoning occurs, the digestive tract plays an important role in eliminating the poison, by ejecting it from the system as quickly as possible. It does this by expelling the food from either the top or bottom of the tract by vomiting or diarrhoea. Less drastic symptoms of food poisoning include milder forms of indigestion, such as irritation of the mucous membranes, causing discomfort in the throat and/or the stomach, and feelings of nausea.

There are plenty of natural toxins in food that, in small amounts, we deal with effectively without suffering adverse effects. Ingesting them in large amounts, however, is a different matter. Solanine – the substance in green potatoes – is one such example.

Potatoes normally contain about 7 mg of solanine per 100-g (4-oz) serving. It is found mostly in green skin, but also in the eyes and sprouts of potatoes. It isn't enough just to cut off the green bits and remove the eyes, as the solanine can spread throughout the potato. When very small amounts of solanine are eaten, mild forms of poisoning occur that manifest themselves as general gastrointestinal discomfort, such as stomach ache and aches in the intestines, too. As the levels of solanine consumed rise, symptoms of nausea, vomiting and diarrhoea quickly set in. If levels of 33 mg per 100 g are reached, trouble really starts as the nervous system then becomes affected, with fever and the risk of circulatory collapse.

It is best to avoid potatoes with any sign of greening or sprouting. Always store them in a cool, dry, dark place to reduce the risk of solanine being produced, which happens when they are exposed to light for more than just a few days.

Toxins in poisonous mushrooms are another cause of vomiting and diarrhoea. *Amanita phalloides* is the mushroom most commonly responsible for poisoning in Britain. If only small amounts are ingested, you may get away with just abdominal pain.

Problems with mussels infected with saxitoxin are more likely than finding a rogue mushroom in your food, as there is no way of telling whether or not the mussel on your plate has fed on plankton containing the saxitoxin. Mussels themselves are not affected by it and, as it is not killed by cooking, it is only after eating a 'bad' one that you know because then you will be suffering from severe vomiting and diarrhoea.

As well as naturally occurring toxins, normally healthy foods and drinks can become infected by bacteria, which, once eaten, affect the digestive tract. Bacteria such as salmonella infect the intestines directly, causing upsets and aches, whereas others produce toxins and it is these toxins that do the damage, such as clostridium. The symptoms may be very severe and obviously linked to something recently consumed. Equally likely, however, are much milder levels of infection and these lead to general discomfort in the stomach and gut, feelings of nausea, queasiness and general indigestion, which won't be attributed to food poisoning.

Problems with food poisoning have always existed. The processing food undergoes now in the West attempts to reduce the risk by using a variety of techniques, such as pasteurization, canning and cooking, which all act as safeguards. The storage and handling of food and drink by the industry, retailer and ourselves at home play vital roles in keeping food poisoning under control.

Common Forms of Food Poisoning
Bacterial

Salmonella

Salmonella is the name given to a group of bacteria, of which there are more than 1,600 types. They are among the most common causes of food poisoning, infecting poultry and many other intensively reared animals. When we eat the infected meat, the bacteria are taken in with the food and usually stay in the intestinal tract where they wreak their havoc, causing pain, diarrhoea and vomiting. This usually begins around 12 to 36 hours after having eaten the contaminated food. It is quite common to be able to trace the symptoms back to a certain meal by checking how the people you ate with are feeling, as it is likely that all the people who ate the same food will be similarly affected. The digestive problems will usually last for up to two to three days.

Most cases of salmonella occur as a result of uncooked or badly cooked foods, or food that has been cooked and recontaminated. If, for example, an egg custard pie is cut with a knife that has been used for raw poultry and not thoroughly washed before being used again, the egg custard could easily become infected.

People can become carriers of salmonella. They have salmonella but don't have any symptoms, yet can pass the bacteria on to infect and affect others.

Basic Rules for Avoiding Salmonella Contamination

Meat and meat products, poultry, eggs, milk and milk products are the foods most commonly susceptible to salmonella contamination. If they are stored, handled and prepared properly, they do not pose a risk.

● When storing uncooked poultry, it should be kept in a fridge at less than 5°C and in a container that will not allow juices to drip on to foods below.

- Food should always be prepared with clean equipment and this should be thoroughly washed afterwards.

- Food should be cooked for long enough and at the correct temperatures.

- Cracked or damaged eggs should not be used and neither should those past the sell-by date. Dirty eggs should be wiped with a dry, clean cloth, but not washed as this destroys the protective film.

- Unpasteurized milk should be avoided.

Campylobacter

Stomach pains and discomfort followed by diarrhoea and fever are common symptoms of infection with campylobacter. The main type to infect the digestive system is *Campylobacter jejuni*. They are present in foods such as raw milk, some raw meats and poultry and unchlorinated water supplies. Campylobacter do not multiply in food, but once they enter the stomach and gut, they feed on what is for them a nutritionally rich medium that has the requisite low oxygen content and multiply with great speed. The symptoms are seldom serious and it is possible that an unexplained bout of indigestion could be down to mild infections with this bacteria.

The best way to avoid such infection is to consume only pasteurized or UHT milk, only drink water from known sources and avoid cross-contamination between cooked and uncooked foods. Heating does kill the bacteria, so cooked foods eaten hot are usually no problem.

Escherichia Coli

Consuming food or drink infected with *Escherichia coli* (usually simply *E. coli*) will again adversely affect the digestive tract. When the bacteria are ingested, they sit in the intestines and produce toxins, which lead to stomach pains, diarrhoea and maybe vomiting, too. The illness can last from one to seven days. Mild forms may cause cramps and indigestion that does not lead on to severe symptoms.

E. coli live in the large intestine and are transferred to food by means of poor personal hygiene. Simply thoroughly washing hands after going to the toilet and drying them on a clean towel is the best way of stopping them spreading. Meat can be infected with *E. coli* from humans or other animals. Care in handling is therefore vital to prevent infection.

Staphylococcus Aureus

Digestive tract symptoms of infection with *S. aureus* are similar to other types of food poisoning, including stomach cramps, nausea, diarrhoea and vomiting. The uppermost part of the digestive tract can also be affected, with excess saliva being produced. The bacteria produce a toxin that takes effect one to four hours after eating and can last for up to two days. *S. aureus* are found in the nasal passages of humans and animals and also often found in infected wounds and boils. They can also be passed from infected cattle into their milk.

As with *E. coli*, good hygiene can help avoid infections. Keeping hands clean and covering cuts and wounds is essential. Once the toxins have been produced, they cannot be destroyed by heating so preventing them from contaminating the food in the first place is vital. Poultry, meat, fish, milk and milk products are most susceptible to contamination with this bacteria.

Bacillus Cereus

If you become infected with *Bacillus cereus*, you will know about it all too soon. Usually within an hour, the bacteria have produced a toxin that will bring about waves of nausea and general discomfort in the stomach. If the poisoning is bad, sickness will follow within an hour and diarrhoea will start after eight hours.

B. cereus is found in the soil, but can find its way into the food chain. Once in food, the bacteria produce a toxin that actually only does the damage when the food is eaten. Boiled and fried rice are foods commonly affected by this bacteria, especially if cooked in bulk and left to stand for some time at normal room temperature. Custards, cereal products, puddings and sauces can also be affected.

The best way to avoid infection with *B. cereus* is to chill foods as quickly as possible once they have been cooked. Large quantities should be divided up into smaller amounts to speed up cooling and then be stored in the fridge. If reheated, it should be to temperatures above 70°C.

Moulds

Moulds are part of the fungi group of organisms. Most moulds are white and look furry or fuzzy, like fine cotton wool, although some are dark or coloured. Eating mouldy foods can upset the stomach and lead to vomiting and sickness.

Moulds usually turn foods bad and some also produce mycotoxins, which will cause harm when eaten. Some, however, are used in the food industry to make, for example, soy sauce and blue cheeses.

Mouldy foods should be thrown away. Scraping it off does not remove any toxins that may have been produced and have entered the food. Moulds are spread in the air as tiny spores that land on a food and multiply rapidly, which is another good reason for not disturbing it by cutting, but simply throw the whole piece away.

─── 8 ───
Cleansing and Calming the Gut Naturally

Self-cleansing of the gut does not require you to book an appointment for colonic irrigation. Manually evacuating the bowel disturbs the natural balance of bacteria which have built themselves up in the large intestine, and is generally regarded at best with scepticism by gastroenterologists, and at worst as a harmful practice.

This chapter on self-cleansing and calming is about learning how to take control of your digestive system and being kind to it. You can do this through ensuring your regular diet is well suited to your own particular digestive make-up, and by employing the use of herbs, supplements and foods with added ingredients designed specifically to improve intestinal health. It is also about taking time out to relax, de-stress and get yourself into good emotional shape.

The need to cleanse and calm the digestive system is nothing new. Since we first started roaming the planet, humans have been seeking the means by which to maintain and restore balance to their sensitive intestines. If you put together, in any combination, the potent forces of food, drink, overindulgence, intolerances, stress and anxiety, it's easy enough to work out why. Since digestive complaints are nothing new, it's not surprising that herbal medicine, which has been practised since time immemorial, has many remedies at its fingertips.

In addition to herbal solutions, basic good nutrition has a vital role to play in the repair and maintenance of the system. Some modern medical approaches to digestive problems also have their place.

Before trying any self-help or over-the-counter medications, check out your symptoms with your doctor to ensure your problems do not need medical or surgical intervention.

Cleansing

Water

Crucial to a healthy, cleansed gut is an adequate daily intake of water. You need it to digest food, dissolve nutrients so that they can pass through the intestinal cell walls into your bloodstream, and move food through the intestinal tract. Inadequate water can lead to constipation, especially when combined with a high-fibre diet. When the large intestine slows down its slow rhythmic movements, the bowel contents have the chance to stay in contact with the bowel wall for greater lengths of time, allowing potential toxins and cancer-causing substances to take a foothold. Looser, faster-moving, well-hydrated stools decrease the chances of this happening and thus reduce the risk of subsequent diseases whether they are infectious toxins or carcinogenic in origin.

Since the body does not have the ability to store water, a new supply must be taken daily, and this must be enough to replace losses from breath and perspiration (850–1,200 ml/30–42 fl oz), urination (600–1,600 ml/21–56 fl oz) and that lost through the stools (50 – 200 ml/2–7 fl oz): a grand total of 1½ —3 litres (3–6 US pints) of water a day.

Some of this water we get through food, but it is wise to try to drink around 2–2½ litres (4–5 US pints) a day. Bear in mind that not all liquids are equally liquefying. The caffeine in tea and coffee and the alcohol in alcoholic drinks have a diuretic effect, which makes you urinate more and thus lose some of the benefits of the liquid part of the drink.

People who eat a lot of salt and those taking exercise need to increase fluid intakes. After an hour's exercise you can lose a good litre (35 fl oz) of body water through perspiration. It is important to keep drinking throughout the day. Remember, by the time your mouth is dry and you are registering thirst, you are already dehydrated.

If you become dehydrated through lack of access to fluids or perhaps through diarrhoea, the quickest way to rehydrate is with isotonic sports drinks such as Lucozade Sport or Gatorade. You can make your own version by taking a glass of squash or concentrated fruit juice and adding a pinch of salt.

Probiotics

Altering the balance of undesirable bacteria in favour of the health-enhancing varieties is a concept with which we are becoming familiar. This cleansing of the large intestine from the inside out is a growing market with more and more products, most of which are milk- and dairy-based, on supermarket shelves. 'Live yogurts' have made their way out of the specialist health food stores and now sit proudly alongside established brands. We even see little Japanese fermented milk available by the tills of the local shop.

The key to an effective probiotic is knowing that the bacteria can survive the acidic stomach environment, the alkaline conditions of the duodenum, and be able to make it to the large intestine. Few in practice are able to do this. Once in the bowel, the probiotic needs to be able to attach itself to the wall and successfully reproduce.

Intensive research carried out in Sweden has shown that five of the 20 or so different strains of *Lactobacilli* bacteria which are commonly present in the intestine have this ability. Scientists have proved that of these five, *Lactobacillus plantarum* 299v adheres particularly well to the intestinal wall and reduces the number of anaerobic bacteria and toxin-producing clostridia which are particularly problematic in the gut. *Lactobacillus plantarum* 299v helps to cleanse and rebalance the gut after courses of antibiotics, chronic diarrhoea, inflammatory intestinal diseases, cramps and post-operative infections. It can also be taken on a daily basis as a protective measure. This unique and effective probiotic is available in a fruit juice-based drink known as Proviva. Being non-dairy, it is the first effective probiotic available to those who are milk-intolerant.

Soluble and Insoluble Fibre

There cannot be a more natural way of spring cleaning your digestive tract than increasing your intake of fibrous foods. Starting in the mouth, foods rich in fibre give the teeth and gums a physical workout. Once in the stomach, both soluble fibrous fractions (found in oats, beans, apples and pears) and insoluble fractions (in wholegrain cereals and some vegetables) can wrap up potential disease-forming substances and sweep them out of the system.

Certain soluble fibres which form gels in the small intestine can bind bacteria to them so that both leave the gut via the stools. Insoluble fibres, on the other hand, literally absorb potentially harmful cancer-inducing substances. They do so by binding water to their surface and trapping the baddies within the bulky stools. Fibre is also capable of diluting carcinogens lurking within the colonic contents and moving them swiftly out of the gut.

Nourishing the Tract Itself

Since the digestive tract is surrounded for its entire length by muscles, not surprisingly nutrients which feed and nurture muscular tissue are important to the system's ability to keep moving at the correct pace. Equally, vitamins and minerals that are essential for the correct functioning of the nerves and hormones which regulate muscle movement must be supplied in adequate amounts if the system is to keep moving.

A diet rich in carbohydrates, as found in bread, cereals, rice, pasta, potatoes and fruits, provides muscles with a constant source of energy in the form of glucose and the stored form of glucose, glycogen. Dairy products, nuts, seeds, dark green vegetables and dried fruits supply both calcium and magnesium, minerals needed by muscle fibres to contract and relax, thus creating the peristaltic waves which move the digested food contents along.

For the nervous system, a good and constant supply of B vitamins are needed, especially B_6 (in meat, milk and potatoes) and B_{12} (in meat, dairy products, fish, eggs and fortified soya milks and breakfast cereals). Folic acid is also important, and can be found in wholegrain cereals, fortified breads and cereals and Marmite (yeast extract).

Herbal Cleansers

Herbs can provide a simple yet effective way of cleansing various parts of the digestive system.

The Mouth

For cleansing the mouth, try adding 5 ml (about 1 teaspoonful) of myrrh tincture to a glass of warm water and use as a mouthwash to benefit from its antimicrobial properties. A similar quantity of bistort tincture can be added to water for an astringent cleanse, or try 10 ml of sage tincture diluted in water – this has antiseptic qualities and is thus good for helping fight gum disorders and gingivitis.

The Large Intestine

To lubricate and bulk the bowel contents to help flush them through, try infusing a teaspoon of psyllium seeds or linseeds in a cup of boiling water. Allow them to cool and drink with the seeds twice daily. To speed gut contents, take 2 ml of rhubarb tincture three times a day. The antraquinones in the rhubarb irritate the gut lining and increase its movements.

Sorbitol is a sugar alcohol found in some fruits, such as plums, apricots, cherries and apples. It is made for commercial use from fruit sugars and is added to many sugar-free products. Sorbitol is absorbed quite slowly from the intestine and tends to draw water into it. If eaten in large amounts – a tube of sugar-free mints in one sitting, for example – it can stimulate bowel contractions and lead to a fast clear-out of the colon contents.

The same is true of prunes, which contain derivatives of a substance called hydroxyphenylizaton that directly stimulates the smooth muscle of the colon wall.

Other foods which have this natural laxative effect include rhubarb, figs, liquorice, molasses, senna and castor oil.

Nurturing
The Gut Lining

Keeping the lining of the digestion system in good condition from the mouth right down to the rectum and anus is important for many reasons, from helping to prevent mouth ulcers to stopping the colon becoming 'leaky' and thus allowing dangerous bacteria to move from the tract into the blood and set up life-threatening infections in other organs.

Vitamin A, as found in liver (not suitable for pregnant women), whole dairy products, eggs, carrots and dark green vegetables, and vitamin E as found in wheatgerm, avocados and nuts, are both needed for membrane health. So too are the essential fatty acids (EFAs) found in oily fish, flax seed oil and evening primrose oil.

To soothe an irritated stomach lining you need to avoid foods and drinks which increase stomach acid secretion. These include alcohol, caffeine and hot spicy foods. Try a tincture of meadowsweet or liquorice, both of which are anti-inflammatory. The former soothes and heals the stomach lining while the latter helps to produce a viscous mucus which coats the stomach wall and reduces acid secretion.

An inflamed lining can also be helped by the essential fatty acids in fish and evening primrose oil, which both act by sup-pressing the pro-inflammatory substances.

For the large intestine, regularly taking probiotics (see page 71) strengthens the gut wall bacteria and allows them to fight off potentially dangerous invaders.

Enzyme Release

For the intestine to carry out its primary function of digesting and absorbing foods, the enzymes which do the physical breaking down need to be in plentiful supply and their secretion under proper control. Zinc from red meats and wholegrain foods, magnesium from milk products, selenium from brazil nuts, cereals and fish, and copper from wholemeal bread and vegetables are all important for the activation of these enzymes.

Calming

The tremendous effects (both perceptible and imperceptible) which the nerves surrounding the intestines and those in the central nervous system have on the physical functioning of the digestive tract should never be underestimated. When you have been through or find yourself experiencing a stressful period in your life, then you can be sure that your gut will feel the effects. To calm things down there is much that can be done, both by turning to the world of herbs and looking at alternative forms of exercise and meditation.

Herbal Helpers

For general anxiety and tension an infusion, tincture or capsules of skullcap are often recommended by herbalists. Infusions or tinctures of linden or vervain may also prove useful. To aid relaxation, tinctures of mugwort, gotu kola, lavender or camomile can be taken. Lemon balm tea and valerian tablets offer another option.

Alternative Therapies for Calming the Nervous System

Acupuncture

Originating in China, acupuncture is based on the concept that disease involves an imbalance within the body systems. Treatment is intended to restore equilibrium and balance; it is achieved by inserting appropriate needles in exactly the right places (along points known as meridians) by the practitioners. The nervous system is said to respond well to this form of treatment. Usually within seconds of the needles being positioned, a deeply relaxed – even drowsy – state is experienced. For the most part acupuncture in the UK is not available on the NHS and you will need to find a qualified, private practitioner should you wish to try this therapy.

Aromatherapy

This makes use of a combination of body and face massage using essential oils extracted from plants. It can be practised as an extension of herbalism or simply as part of a beauty massage. In aromatherapy it is the aromatic oils which give plants their distinctive smells (the essences) that are used. These can come from the roots, flowers, leaves, bark or resin, and no two are alike. In the plants themselves these essences serve particular functions such as acting as pesticides, fungicides and bactericides, and are often used in the cosmetics and toiletries we use daily. Aroma-therapists use these essences, massaging them into the skin. These essences then make their way into the body's extra-cellular fluids.

Oils of melissa and rosemary have a calming effect when used in a specific dose. For nervous tension, bergamot, camphor, camomile, rose, ylang-ylang, sandalwood and orange blossom are among the first choices. A massage with these oils will prove relaxing and also help calm inner tensions and stress.

Biofeedback Training

This treatment involves training the body to modify specific activities with the benefit of experience. A biofeedback expert can train you to increase particular types of brain waves to make you feel relaxed and pleasant. Biofeedback opens up tremendous scope to us as individuals to control our reactions and moods, especially when we know we are going to be plunged into a stressful situation.

Hypnosis

Hypnosis alters the state of the mind but does *not* send you to sleep. A session of hypnotherapy can leave you deeply relaxed. Direct suggestion therapy is a good place to start.

Massage

Massage in all its forms can have the most tremendously comforting, de-stressing effects on the body. Feeling cosseted, cared for and soothed helps even the most uptight person relax, and leaves a person feeling calm, refreshed and revitalized.

There are many different types of massage techniques, one of which is bound to suit you as an individual. You could, for example, try Reiki, for which the practitioner has been attuned to act as a channel for 'Ki', meaning 'life-force'. Ki is drawn from the masseur's hands to exactly where the recipient needs it, helping to clean the body of toxins and create a state of balance on the physical, emotional and spiritual levels.

Shiatsu is another option. Literally meaning 'finger pressure', it is a form of Japanese massage and pressure designed to stimulate the acupuncture points and meridians. In some ways we all already know about the practice of shiatsu. When a mother rubs a child's bruised leg better or we soothe our own knocks and bumps by rubbing the injured site with our hands, it is the transference of healing powers at work, and this is what shiatsu is all about. A good practitioner can use the technique to calm even the most strung-out individuals.

Yoga

The word yoga means 'oneness' in Sanskrit; it is a personal self-help system for both physical and spiritual health. Learning the postures and breathing techniques can help us unravel many ailments and the emotional knots we tie ourselves up in. With practice it is possible to alter your heart rate and blood pressure and find a wonderful sense of relaxation. Specific postures can actually help to improve ailments of the digestive tract.

Orthodox Remedies for Disturbed Digestion

For the Stomach

Until recently, neutralization of the acidic conditions in the stomach had been the only way to deal with indigestion in this part of the tract, and this method has been used for several centuries. More recently it has been discovered that it is possible to control the actual production of acid in a very specific way. It is also recognized that in addition to controlling the production of acid, it is worth looking into ways of fortifying the usual protective mechanism of the stomach – the mucous membranes.

Controlling the acidity in the stomach is an important part of the treatment for ulcers and severe acid reflux.

Neutralizing Acids – Antacids

Antacid literally means anti-acid, and antacid medicines are designed to neutralize the acid in the stomach. The various ones are therefore made from one or more alkaline substances. Liquid preparations work fastest, but tablets are more convenient to carry around.

By neutralizing the acid in the stomach, antacids produce two desirable effects. They decrease the total amount of acid that moves on into the duodenum and stop the activity of pepsin (one of the enzymes in the stomach juices that breaks down protein). Over long periods, all antacids can have side-effects, so they shouldn't be taken for more than two weeks or so. With those you can buy over the counter at your pharmacist, it is best to check with your doctor before taking them and essential to do so if you are pregnant or breast-feeding, on a low-sodium diet, suffer from heart, blood pressure, liver or kidney problems, or take other medicines on a regular basis.

There are two main types of antacids. Those which are absorbed into the bloodstream and are therefore capable of increasing the pH level of the blood as well as the stomach, which leads to alkaline urine being produced. Then there are the ones that are not absorbed and so do not affect the blood. These are preferable to the absorbed kind if the medicine is to be taken over a couple of weeks.

What is in antacids?

- *Baking soda* Known chemically as sodium bicarbonate or sodium carbonate, these are fast and effective antacids, although they can wear off quickly. They can also lead to belching because they produce carbon dioxide in the stomach. The sodium content makes them out of bounds for anyone with a heart condition, high blood pressure, liver or kidney problems. These antacids are the type that are absorbed into the bloodstream.

- *Chalk* The chemical name for chalk is calcium carbonate. Like baking soda, chalk is an effective antacid. It does release carbon dioxide as it sets to work, however, and can lead to constipation, so it should not be taken for long periods. It is capable of interacting with other medicines like antibiotics, too, so, again, check with your doctor before taking. These antacids are not absorbed into the bloodstream.

- *Aluminium hydroxide* This is less effective than the two above. Like chalk, it has a constipating effect, so it is usually available in a preparation that also contains magnesium, which has a laxative effect so they cancel each other out. This type of antacid must be avoided if you have kidney problems and is known to interact with some antibiotics, antifungal drugs, warfarin and digoxin.

- *Magnesium carbonate, magnesium trisilicate, magnesium hydroxide* These are effective antacids, but they have a laxative effect. They are usually found in combination with calcium or aluminium and are another type that should be avoided if you have kidney problems.

These are the main active ingredients in antacids, but they also contain other ingredients to help relieve various symptoms.

- *Dimethicone or simethicone* This is added to help break up the gas bubbles, although there is little really good evidence regarding its effectiveness. It is supposed to work by allowing the gas bubbles to coalesce (join together) and then be expelled.

- *Alginic acid* This comes from seaweed and, when it reaches the stomach, forms into a foamy gel. This gel works by sitting as a raft on top of the stomach's contents, preventing them from refluxing out of the stomach and back up into the oesophagus.

Antacids are useful for helping ulcers to heal, if taken properly. Their disadvantage is that they have to be taken regularly and, as mentioned, have side-effects. The chalky taste most of them have is often poorly accepted, which means that people tend to stop taking them before they have had their beneficial effect and healing has been completed. It would seem that antacids are not as safe as some of the newer treatments, which actually stop the acid being produced in the first place.

Blocking Acid Production

How acid is produced and secreted into the stomach was described earlier, but, to refresh our memories, it is controlled by several mechanisms.

1. Nerve stimulation, which can be triggered by the sight, smell and taste of food and its arrival in the stomach. The particular nerve involved is the vagus nerve, which releases a substance called acetycholine and this fixes on to a special receptor site in the acid-secreting parietal cells in the stomach wall. This action then stimulates acid secretion.

2. By a hormone called gastrin. Gastrin is released from the mucous membranes of the stomach when food is present. The gastrin latches on to its own special gastrin receptor sites in the parietal cell to stimulate acid secretion.

3. By the action of a substance called histamine, which itself is stimulated by the presence of food in the stomach and by acetylcholine and gastrin. Histamine latches on to a histamine receptor in the acid-secreting parietal gland.

When just one of these three stimulators fixes on to the parietal cell, the secretion of acid is scanty. When all three fix on to it, though, the acid literally pours into the stomach.

Mechanisms to reduce acid secretion therefore involve blocking the substances that cause the parietal cells to release it. These are the following.

Anticholinergics

These drugs stop the impulses from the vagus nerve getting to the acid-secreting cells in the stomach wall. They are able to reduce acid secretion but do not stop it completely.

Anticholinergics were known to have various side-effects. For example, some people found they developed blurred vision, others developed a dry mouth, making chewing and swallowing difficult. Small doses may still be used, but, in the main, they have been replaced by the following more modern treatments.

H₂ Antagonists

These substances are able to latch on to the histamine receptor site on the parietal cell and effectively prevent the histamine latching on. If no histamine is locked on to the receptor, the parietal cell will not release any acid. It's rather like blocking someone's keyhole up with filler or glue – there is then no way for them to get their key into the door and thus turn it to enter. H_2 receptor blockers, or antagonists, as they are called, include substances with names like famotidine, cimetidine and ranitidine and block all three stimulators of the acid-secreting cell.

H_2 blockers work by reducing the background level of acid during the day and night in the stomach, as well as the amount of acid that is released during the day in response to eating and drinking, and even just thinking about food. The decrease in acid secretion that results from this blocking allows the mucous membranes, in particular the duodenal ones, to tolerate the lower acidity of the material it receives from the stomach, which gives the ulcer a better chance of healing, improves the speed at which healing occurs and helps prevent the recurrence of ulcers.

Side-effects of these medicines are usually rare and minor, although people with kidney problems do need to take them in lower doses. There can also be interaction with other medication, like warfarin, so, again, care needs to be taken.

The H_2 receptor sites are not the same as the histamine receptor sites in the airways and air passages – these are H_1 sites. These are not therefore affected by the H_2 antagonist drugs used to treat indigestion.

Proton Pump Inhibitors

Once the sites on the parietal cell have been locked on to, whether it is by acetylcholine, gastrin or histamine, all then go on to cause hydrochloric acid to be secreted into the stomach by a pump action. There is a group of drugs that can interfere with this final part of the process so that even if the receptor sites have been stimulated, acid production can still be stopped. These drugs are called proton pump inhibitors.

They produce a more rapid response and promote a faster rate of healing of ulcers than H_2 antagonists and are particularly good for people suffering from refluxing up into the throat or oesophagus. They can, however, cause side-effects, including headaches, rashes and diarrhoea.

Antibiotics

Since the emergence of the theory that stomach ulcers may be caused by the bacteria *Helicobacter pylori* (*H. pylori*), many doctors now treat stomach and duodenal ulcers with a cocktail of drugs. Such a cocktail would include an antibiotic, taken for a week or two, to eradicate the bacteria, and an H_2 blocker, such as cimetidine, famotidine or ranitidine to control acid secretion and give the ulcerated region a chance to heal. Such treatment seems to work very effectively.

Mucus-protecting Agents

Another group of substances can help, too – the cytoprotectants. They act by increasing the secretion of the protective mucus and bicarbonate, and/or by actually providing a physical barrier, thus covering up the ulcer, preventing further irritation of the area to aid healing.

Sucralfate, for example, is thought to act by coating the ulcer, by forming a sticky substance which protects against acid, pepsin and bile salts. It also stimulates the production of mucus, bicarbonate and prostaglandins. It is effective in helping the healing of ulcers.

Another long name to remember is carbenoxolone sodium. This helps the healing of gastric and duodenal ulcers along by improving mucosal defence. It is not the usual first choice in ulcer treatment because of the availability of other more modern drugs that have effective track records. Carbenoxolone sodium is not suitable for children, pregnant women, the elderly or those with heart, kidney or liver problems.

Pharmacy Availability of H₂ Blockers

Doctors have been able to prescribe H$_2$ blockers for some years. Some well-known ones are Tagamet (cimetidine), Zantac (ranitidine) and Pepcid (famotidine). However, it is now possible to buy weaker versions from the chemists as an 'over-the-counter' product – in other words, you ask the pharmacist for it. The pharmacist should run through a checklist before allowing you to have it, though, to check that it is safe for you to take.

—— 9 ——
You're Not Alone

If you suffer with digestive problems then you most definitely are not alone. In the UK alone around 14 million people at any one time are experiencing problems with bloating, aching, bouts of wind and general discomfort. These problems can disrupt pleasure and leisure time, work, sleep and the ability to enjoy food and drink.

One of the largest surveys carried out to discover more about such complaints questioned 1,004 people to gain an insight into causes and how people deal with their problems. Men and women, it was discovered, suffer in equal amounts and no age group remained untouched by symptoms, although people between the ages of 35 and 64 were the most affected. Those in professional occupations were most prone to attacks, followed by managerial and manual workers. Of all the people questioned, 80 per cent could relate their digestive problems to a particular cause.

Problem Foods

The foods listed here were those perceived to provoke negative digestive reactions.

- fatty foods, 58 per cent
- spicy foods, 47 per cent
- alcohol, 39 per cent
- fizzy drinks, 37 per cent
- rich foods, 31 per cent
- onions, 29 per cent
- peppers, 24 per cent

- citrus fruits, 23 per cent
- fruit juice, 20 per cent
- garlic, 17 per cent
- tomatoes, 13 per cent
- chocolate, 13 per cent
- coffee, 12 per cent
- food containing air, 9 per cent
- cabbage, 6 per cent.

Women seemed to be more aware of which particular types of foods triggered their indigestion than were men. Fatty foods, for example, were more frequently pinpointed by women than men. Spicy foods, second on the list, were, again, mentioned more often by women than men.

Alcohol and fizzy drinks came next. Alcohol was the second most common cause stated by men, and, in fact, the only factor mentioned significantly more often by men than women. The difficulties caused by alcohol follow the general trends seen in alcohol consumption. Men and those in work mentioned this cause more often than other groups. The older respondents had less trouble with alcohol sparking off indigestion, which is in line with the general drop in alcohol consumption in this group.

Rich foods were unspecified but acknowledged by a significant number of the people asked to be a contributing factor to their digestive upsets.

Among the individual foods mentioned, onions and peppers were the most frequently pinpointed. The survey revealed that indigestion following eating citrus fruit was more of a problem in older people and they mentioned fruit juices as a cause more often, too. Less frequently mentioned were problems triggered by garlic, tomatoes, chocolate and coffee. Those who thought eating foods with air in them were to blame named popcorn and meringues as potential causes.

The people taking part in the survey were then asked what they avoided because it gave them indigestion. The answers they gave are shown below in perceived order of importance.

Factor	Percentage who avoided it
Overeating/eating too quickly	85
Stress	59
Putting on weight	58
Eating before bed	58
Exercising after meals	55
Tight clothing	51
Eating fast foods	49
Smoking	31
Bending	30

Stress

Of the people taking part in the survey, almost 60 per cent said that stress played a big role in digestive upsets. Family problems lay at the heart of many of the cases. For women, juggling the commitments of children, elderly relatives, holding down a job and coping with family life were triggers. Adjusting lifestyles was one of the key factors they felt needed addressing. Take a look at some of the suggestions in Chapter 7 to help you take control and make changes to your current way of life.

Other Factors

Overeating and eating too rapidly were other key areas which people identified as being a source of their digestive turmoil. Wearing tight clothes, laying down after eating and pregnancy were also said to be triggers. Clearly these are all things which can be addressed by the individual. Making time for meals and snacks is crucial. Try planning ahead and giving yourself, at the very least, five minutes each side of eating. Keep your tight clothes for special occasions, and avoid wearing them when you know you will be expected to eat a large meal.

Self-Help

Keeping symptoms to ourselves seems to be one of the key features of digestive disorders. Most people seem to find ways of coping without making a fuss. Some turn to orthodox treatments and do not make any attempt to change eating habits or lifestyles, while others take positive steps to get to the root of the problem. It is crucial that before turning to the kind of solutions outlined in the case histories below, that you first consult with your doctor so that he or she can rule out any underlying problems which need to be dealt with through medical or surgical intervention.

Caroline, 32: Stress-related Stomach Cramps

A fashion buyer for a large chain store, Caroline works long hours at an unrelentingly fast pace. Her job demands a lot of travel and out-of-hours entertaining.

'I suppose my digestive system is uptight from the moment I open my eyes in the morning. I know the rushed feeling must get transferred to all my internal organs including my stomach. I don't have breakfast because the butterfly feeling stops me wanting to eat, and whenever I do have something, experience tells me I rush it down and feel uncomfortable for the rest of the morning. The same pretty much goes for lunch, a bolted sandwich seems to give me stomach cramps, pain and bloating, so unless I'm with clients it's usually just a piece of fruit which I grab on the go. Dinner is usually at a restaurant where most of the foods on offer are rich, and if I'm feeling nervous about the people I'm dining with because they are important to business then I know I'll pay for my meal with a bad stomach later.

'I can honestly say the only time I enjoy food is at the weekend when I can eat the foods I enjoy and do so at my own pace. I know that there is nothing seriously wrong with me, partly because my doctor told me so but more because I feel fine when I'm able to relax. I was advised by a friend to start taking yoga classes so that I could learn how to breathe in a controlled way which helps to lower your

heart rate. It's not easy but I am gradually getting the hang of it. If I remember to take five minutes to calm down before a lunch I think my stomach seems to cope better. It's a bit like massaging out a taut muscle, I suppose. It's the only solution I can think of because I certainly don't want to change my job.'

Jenny, 35: Yeast and Sugar Intolerance-induced Bloating, Wind and Thrush

A television executive with a five-year history of thrush and digestive complaints, Jenny finally discovered she was intolerant to sugar and yeast. Diet was the key to her recovery.

'I kept getting bouts of thrush due to a problem with Candida. It was really getting me down and I was fed up with taking medicine which didn't seem to knock it out. It was this which finally led my doctor to refer me to a dietitian, who helped me look at things with a fresh perspective. I was surprised at how draconian her advice was, but I decided that I had better give it a try. She literally made me stop eating all foods containing yeast, which included everything from bread and wine to less obvious things like grapes and plums, cheese, crumpets and even cream crackers. I also had to give up all sugar – and I mean all sugar. I couldn't believe that here was a dietitian telling me not to eat fruit! The diet was difficult to follow and I lapsed a few times. However, my thrush really did start to go. Not only that, the dreadful bloating and wind which I had thought was just a part of everyday life also started to subside.

'I am not as strict about sugar now but I still avoid eating too many yeast-containing foods. I can cope with the odd glass of wine and about two slices of toast a day. I know my limits and I really do stay within them.'

Elizabeth, 54: Irritable Bowel Following Hysterectomy

Elizabeth, an active and sociable housewife, had a hysterectomy when she was 52 and within weeks was suffering bowel symptoms she had never previously experienced.

'I was expecting to feel weak and under the weather for a while after my operation, but to my surprise it wasn't the actual hysterectomy which caused a lot of pain, rather the odd way my bowels started to behave. It was about six weeks after the surgery, during which time I was taking antibiotics for an infection. Quite out of the blue I noticed terrible swings between going to the loo far more often than normal and not going for days on end. The bloating was also bad, but I put this down to the operation.

'I was sent to see a specialist in Irritable Bowel Syndrome, who talked about it being related to emotional problems. I had to be quite tough with him and insisted I was not about to have a breakdown and that I was completely happy with my husband. We don't have any real worries, so eventually he ruled that out. I think he was just testing me out, because very soon after he turned to what I ate and asked me about my favourite foods. I eat a lot of dairy products and bread.

'It was the bread which struck a chord with him. He explained that sometimes the foods we like most can be responsible for changes in bowel habits. That this started after my hysterectomy apparently is not uncommon. It is something to do with the drugs I took and possibly the body's reaction to the whole process of being interfered with.

'Anyway, I've been avoiding wheat in bread but also have had to give up cakes and biscuits, some breakfast cereals and even pies and pasta. Everything is a lot better so it has been worth it, although at times I have felt really rude saying no all the time to the things I love eating when I'm at other people's houses or out to dinner in a nice restaurant.'

Tony, 29: Constant Problems with Heartburn

Tony's job as a taxi driver means he is sitting down virtually all day and gets very little exercise. He eats his lunch on the hoof, grabbing fast foods where and when he gets the chance. His weight has been increasing since he gave up sports and started cabbing.

'Some days I don't know how I kept going. I used to eat a constant supply of mints to keep that acidy feeling out of my throat, and chewed those antacid things like they were going out of fashion. It didn't get any better, though, and there were moments when the pain got so bad I thought I was having a heart attack. The doctor, like my wife, kept on at me to lose weight. He said that the weight, combined with sitting down all day, was the cause of the problem. I'm 17 stone (238 lb) and 5'10", so I'm on the hefty side for someone my age.

'In the end I joined weight watchers. I've heard all the jokes but it is working. I've learned about various foods I can eat plenty of, and various ones I need to be strict with. My wife gives me stuff to take with me and I've knocked the burgers and what-not on the head. Eventually she also persuaded me to see this friend of hers who's into herbs. I've got these little brown bottles of potions we keep in the fridge, and I even drink camomile tea. To be honest the acidy feeling is going. If you'd told me a few years ago that shifting some weight and taking a few herbs could help, I'd have laughed. I thought the old heartburn was my lot in life. Something I had to get used to. It wasn't. I'm beating it and I'm happy about that.'